Dysphagia Evaluation and Treatment

Eiichi Saitoh • Kannit Pongpipatpaiboon
Yoko Inamoto • Hitoshi Kagaya
Editors

Dysphagia Evaluation and Treatment

From the Perspective of Rehabilitation Medicine

Springer

Editors
Eiichi Saitoh
Department of Rehabilitation Medicine I,
School of Medicine, Fujita Health
University
Toyoake, Aichi
Japan

Yoko Inamoto
Faculty of Rehabilitation, School of
Health Sciences, Fujita Health
University
Toyoake, Aichi
Japan

Kannit Pongpipatpaiboon
Department of Rehabilitation Medicine I,
School of Medicine, Fujita Health
University
Toyoake, Aichi
Japan

Hitoshi Kagaya
Department of Rehabilitation Medicine I,
School of Medicine, Fujita Health
University
Toyoake, Aichi
Japan

ISBN 978-981-10-5031-2 ISBN 978-981-10-5032-9 (eBook)
https://doi.org/10.1007/978-981-10-5032-9

Library of Congress Control Number: 2017954327

Printed on acid-free paper

This Springer imprint is published by Springer Nature
The registered company is Springer Nature Singapore Pte Ltd.
The registered company address is: 152 Beach Road, #21-01/04 Gateway East, Singapore 189721, Singapore

Foreword

Dysphagia is a common and potentially serious problem, especially in neurological disorders, and is particularly frequent in elderly individuals. Dysphagia is associated with significant morbidity and mortality including dehydration, malnutrition, airway obstruction, and aspiration pneumonia. Severe dysphagia has a devastating impact on quality of life as it can eliminate the pleasure of eating and drinking. Less recognized is the impact of dysphagia on psychosocial functions. It can lead to isolation as the patient withdraws from activities involving food such as family mealtimes, group dinners, and teatime. These issues are especially important in rapidly aging societies such as Japan, which has the highest percentage of elderly people in the world.

Japan is unique in its early recognition and embrace of the team approach to dysphagia rehabilitation among professionals across a spectrum of disciplines and specialties. Speech language hearing therapists (SHLTs), dentists, nurses, dental hygienists, dieticians, and physiatrists (rehabilitation physicians) actively collaborate in the Japanese dysphagia team. Indeed, the Japanese Society for Dysphagia Rehabilitation is the world's largest multidisciplinary organization dedicated to research, education, and patient care in swallowing disorders. This team approach contributes to both the effectiveness and efficiency of patient care.

Fujita Health University (FHU) is one of the pioneering facilities where dysphagia rehabilitation is approached systematically and scientifically using the concept of the team approach. Their new textbook, *Dysphagia Evaluation and Treatment: From the Perspective of Rehabilitation Medicine*, is designed to support the highest level of practice, scientifically, clinically, and ethically. The chapter authors and editors are highly skilled experts in dysphagia rehabilitation.

I can attest to the exceptional knowledge and expertise of my colleagues at Fujita Health University based on our close and ongoing collaboration since my first visit to Japan in 1996. I have had the good fortune to witness and learn from my colleagues at FHU during many visits to Japan as a visiting professor, especially Professor Eiichi Saitoh, a pioneer and renowned leader in dysphagia research and practice. Additionally, more than 30 Japanese clinicians and researchers have taken research fellowships in my laboratory at Johns Hopkins University, including six current FHU faulty members.

Along with the anatomy and physiology, this textbook highlights basic as well as advanced principles of patient care, including the approach to the patient, bedside examination and screening, instrumental evaluation including traditional as well as novel methods (such as swallowing CT and high resolution manometry), and an approach to treatment based on the science of motor learning. Case studies illustrate the comprehensive team approach to patient care.

This textbook serves as an excellent guide to the latest developments in the practice of dysphagia rehabilitation. This approach, if implemented early and maintained over time, can enhance the health and quality of life of people with dysphagia. It also points the way to improving our knowledge and practice in the future.

Jeffrey B. Palmer, MD
Professor Emeritus, Johns Hopkins University
Baltimore MD 21218, USA
Distinguished Professor, Fujita Health University
Toyoake, Aichi, Japan

Overview

Difficulty swallowing (dysphagia) occurs in all age groups, with a high prevalence in older individuals. The swallowing process requires intricate coordination between the central nervous system and multiple muscles of the face, mouth, pharynx, larynx, and esophagus for safe and effective deglutition. Consequently, dysphagia significantly impacts survival and may become a life-threatening disability.

The older adult population is increasing worldwide. The proportion of individuals ≥60 years of age increased from 9.2% in 1990 to 11.7% in 2013 and is expected to reach 21.1% by 2050 [1]. Japan is at the forefront of the aging population. The older population in Japan is increasing more rapidly than in any of the developed Western European countries or the United States [2]. Japan surpasses all other nations with the highest proportion of older citizens; 26.5% of citizens are >65 years, 12.8% are ≥75 years, and 3.9% are ≥85 years, according to the most recent government statistics in 2015 (final estimates) [3]. Thailand is another Asian country with a growing population of older adults. The number of Thai people aged ≥60 years in 2013 was approximately 9.6 million, accounting for 14% of the population [4]. By 2040, Thailand's older population is expected to increase to 17 million, accounting for 25% of the population [5]. As the older population increases, the incidence of dysphagia associated with the aging process and/or diseases that affect older patients may also increase. For this reason, dysphagia is an increasingly common and concerning problem in Asian societies.

Pneumonia is one of the most common adverse effects of dysphagia and has been a leading cause of death during the past decade. The World Health Organization reported that pneumonia was ranked the fourth leading cause of death worldwide in 2012 (Fig. 1), with a similar trend in Asian countries such as Japan and Thailand (Fig. 2).

Furthermore, pneumonia contributes to increased rates of hospitalization and mortality. The impact of pneumonia in older patients may be more substantial than in other age groups. Data reported by the Nationwide Hospital Admission of

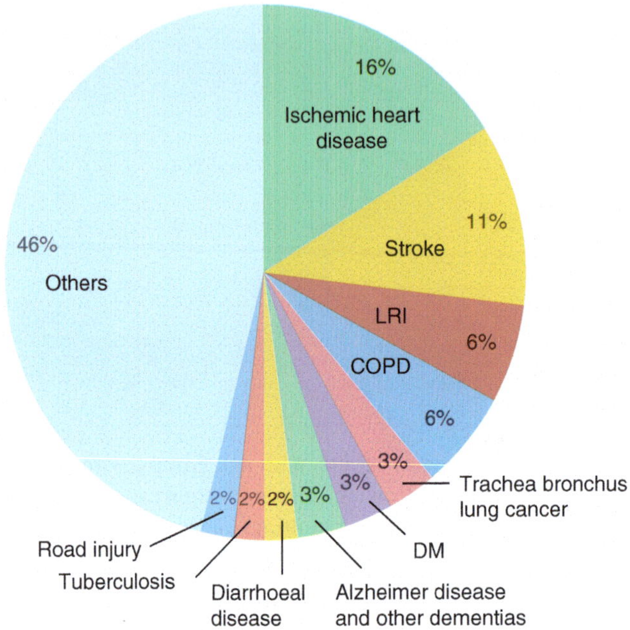

Fig. 1 The 10 leading causes of death worldwide by percentage in 2015 as reported by the World Health Organization. Lower respiratory infections were within the top five leading causes of death worldwide [6]. *COPD* chronic obstructive pulmonary disease, *DM* diabetes mellitus, *LRI* lower respiratory infections

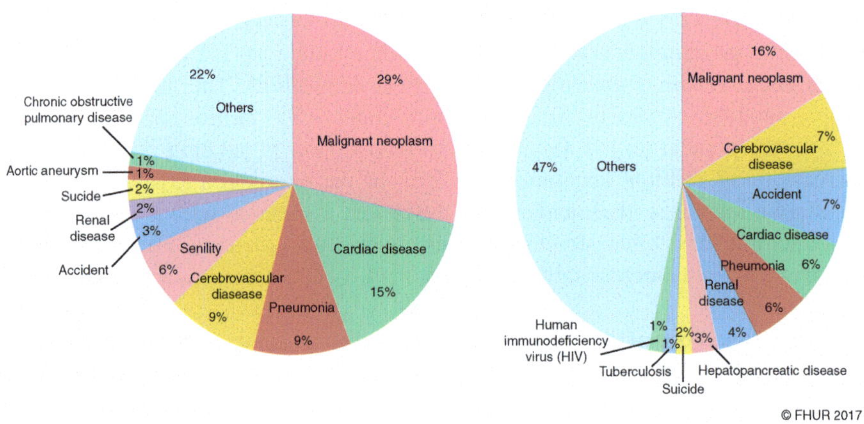

Fig. 2 *Left:* Death rates per 100,000 population by leading cause of death in Japan in 2014 (data derived from the Ministry of Health, Labour and Welfare) [7]. *Right*: Death rates per 100,000 population by leading cause of death in Thailand in 2014 (data derived from the office of the Permanent Secretary for Public Health, Ministry of Public Health) [8]

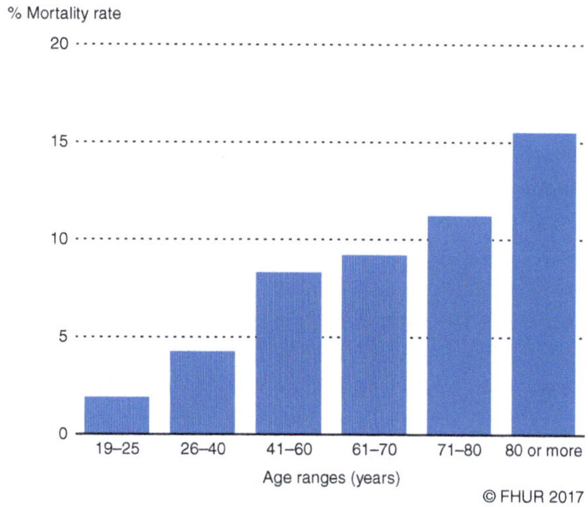

Fig. 3 Increase in pneumonia-associated mortality rate with advancing age in Thailand [9]

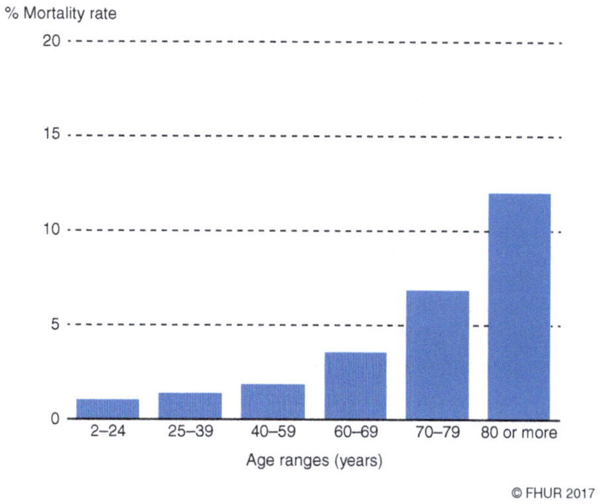

Fig. 4 Increase in pneumonia-associated mortality rate with advancing age in Japan [10]

Thailand in 2010 and a demographic survey performed by the Japanese Ministry of Health, Labour and Welfare in 2015 indicated a rising trend of pneumonia with advancing age and showed a substantially higher mortality rate in afflicted persons aged >60 years (Figs. 3 and 4).

In 2013, a population survey reported by the Japanese Ministry of Health, Labour and Welfare showed that pneumonia was the third leading cause of death overall [7]. Approximately 60% of hospitalized older patients were diagnosed with aspiration pneumonia; this was particularly notable in patients aged ≥70 years [11]. In addition, asphyxiation accounted for the highest proportion of accidental deaths (fifth leading cause of death) in Japan. Many of these patients had dysphagia. These data indicate that dysphagia-related deaths have been increasing and that dysphagia must be thoroughly recognized and understood by healthcare professionals. In 2012, the Fujita Swallowing Team at the Fujita Health University Rehabilitation Complex (FHUR) surveyed the prevalence of dysphagia in Japan and reported 73.7% in chronic hospitals, 59.7% in nursing homes, and 58.7% in long-term care facilities [12]. Similarly, a national survey in 2009 found a relatively large number of geriatric long-term care residents with feeding tubes as well as difficulty swallowing in orally fed residents [13]. This study also indicated that swallowing evaluation in patients with dysphagia is often limited and incomplete [13]. These findings suggest that older residents with dysphagia are not receiving appropriate swallowing evaluation and intervention.

Dysphagia is associated with several problematic outcomes. The severity of dysphagia ranges from mild difficulty to complete inability to swallow and may subsequently give rise to aspiration pneumonia, suffocation, dehydration, malnutrition, and declining quality of life. From the viewpoint of rehabilitation medicine, swallowing is one of the major targets of "activity medicine" (medicine to improve function). Thus, physiatrists and all therapists who play a role in dysphagia management require fundamental knowledge and skills in evaluation and intervention to facilitate safe swallowing and prevent recurrence and other adverse events.

A team approach is indispensable to dysphagia rehabilitation. Interdisciplinary teamwork is a complex process in which staff members from different disciplines work together to share expertise, knowledge, and skills to provide the highest standard of care to patients with dysphagia. Another team approach that involves a joint effort from varying disciplines and is particularly suitable for dysphagia rehabilitation is the transdisciplinary teamwork model. In this model, participating disciplines collaboratively develop a total healthcare plan that addresses all necessary diagnoses and treatments. The Japanese Society of Dysphagia Rehabilitation (JSDR) was founded under the concept of transdisciplinary teamwork [14].

Swallowing teams include specialists from different disciplines, such as physiatrists, dentists, speech-language-hearing therapists, dysphagia-certified nurses, ward nurses, dental hygienists, and dieticians. However, the team may be led by different practitioners based on availability. In Japan, for example, a teamwork-centered approach to dysphagia rehabilitation is emphasized, and speech-language-hearing therapists lead the team in implementing direct and indirect dysphagia training exercises and integrating comprehensive treatment with other disciplines. In other Asian countries, such as Thailand, occupational therapists primarily provide dysphagia rehabilitation services in the form of exercise training regimens for patients with swallowing disorders.

JSDR is a leader in the development and advancement of dysphagia rehabilitation in both clinical and research settings. During the past 20 years, the membership of the JSDR has rapidly risen to more than 11,000 medical professionals (11,653 as of 30 August 2014) from several disciplines (Fig. 5).

Moreover, the JSDR is currently developing relationships with other dysphagia societies in North America, Europe, Asia, and elsewhere across the world to promote international collaboration in the emerging field of deglutition.

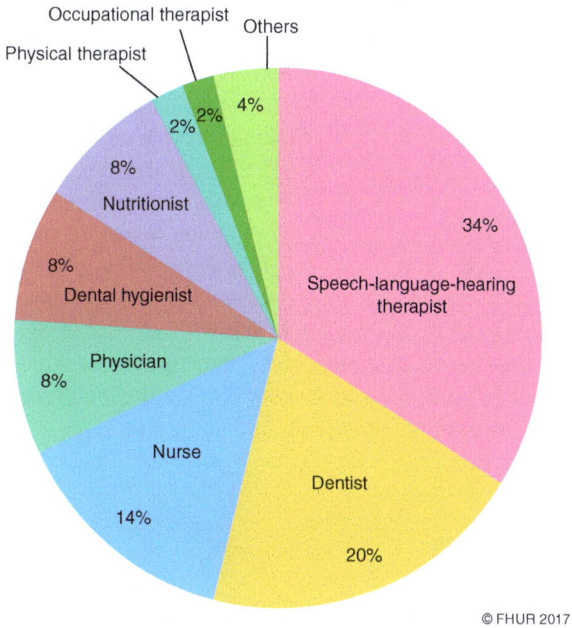

Fig. 5 Disciplines comprising the Japanese Society of Dysphagia Rehabilitation. *DH* dental hygienist, *OT* occupational therapist, *PT* physical therapist, *SLHT* speech-language-hearing therapist

In many Asian countries, dysphagia has become a pressing issue for both physiatrists and rehabilitation therapists. Unfortunately, there may be limited recognition of the prevalence of dysphagia and dysphagia professionals despite the effectiveness of a dysphagia healthcare team. Furthermore, many clinicians are still unfamiliar with dysphagia and lack detailed guidance and practice protocols. Individual clinicians may assess and treat dysphagia differently, complicating research methodology and development of practice consensus. Additionally, patients who present with rare etiologies or subtle signs and symptoms of dysphagia may pose a challenge to clinicians with limited practice.

Instrumental evaluation is necessary to a comprehensive assessment of swallowing of both known and undiagnosed etiologies. Imaging is critical for diagnosing the cause of dysphagia, selecting optimal treatments, and assessing the effects of treatment by accurate measurement of the oropharyngeal swallowing response. The instrumental assessment of dysphagia is a relatively new area of expertise within the field of rehabilitation that has developed over the past several decades in Asian countries. Additionally, considering the shortage of formal dysphagia rehabilitation teams with several specialized clinicians, highly trained professionals are essential for dysphagia management in all settings.

The purpose of this book is to provide all healthcare professionals who are interested in swallowing with the basic practical knowledge required for a broad clinical perspective on dysphagia rehabilitation. This book is neither exhaustive nor encyclopedic; instead, it presents a practical approach to the management and treatment of patients with dysphagia in a real-world clinical setting.

This book is divided into four parts. Part I introduces the general aspects of deglutition and dysphagia with a focus on anatomy and physiology. Part II discusses clinical approaches using both non-instrumental and instrumental evaluation of swallowing. The instrumental evaluations presented include videofluoroscopy, which is considered the gold standard evaluation technique for swallowing disorders, videoendoscopy, and, in brief, 320-row area detector computed tomography, which was recently introduced to analyze three-dimensional swallowing kinematics. Part III addresses the management and treatment of swallowing disorders. Finally, Part IV presents case studies that demonstrate clinical approaches to dysphagia as well as common etiologies encountered in a clinical setting.

The contents of this book follow the model of dysphagia rehabilitation used at FHUR. The Fujita Swallowing Team hopes that it will guide healthcare professionals at all levels and serve as an excellent starting point for the development of expertise in swallowing rehabilitation.

References

1. United Nations, Department of Economic and Social Affairs, Population Division. World Population Ageing 2013. ST/ESA/SER.A/348. 2013.
2. Kuzuya M. Process of physical disability among older adults — contribution of frailty in the super-aged society. Nagoya J Med Sci. 2012;74:31–7.
3. Population estimates by Age. Statistics Bureau, Ministry of Internal Affairs and Communications website. 2015. http://www.stat.go.jp/english/index.htm. Accessed 31 July 2015.
4. Situation of The Thai Elderly 2013, Foundation of Thai Gerontology Research and Development Institute (TGRI). 2013. http://thaitgri.org/?p=37134. Accessed 31 July 2015.
5. UN Department of Economic and Social Affairs, Population Division, 2001, World Population Ageing 1950–2050. 2014. http://ageingasia.org/ageing-population-thailand1/. Accessed 31 July 2015.
6. The World Health Organization (WHO). 2012. http://www.who.int/mediacentre/factsheets/en/. Accessed 24 October 2017.
7. The demographic population survey by Ministry of Health, Labour and Welfare. 2014. http://www.mhlw.go.jp/toukei/saikin/hw/jinkou/geppo/nengai14/dl/gaikyou26.pdf (Japanese). Accessed 31 July 2015.
8. National Statistical Office. Office of the Permanent Secretary for Public Health, Ministry of Public Health, Thailand. 2014. http://www.nso.go.th/ (Thai). Accessed 31 July 2015.
9. Reechaipichitkul W, Thavornpitak Y, Sutra S. Burden of adult pneumonia in Thailand: a nationwide hospital admission data 2010. J Med Assoc Thai. 2014;97(3):283–92.
10. The e-Stat data (an official site of Japanese Government Statistics) by Ministry of Internal Affairs and Communications. http://www.e-stat.go.jp/SG1/estat/List.do?lid=000001137965 (Japanese). Accessed 31 July 2015.

11. Teramoto S, Fukuchi Y, Sasaki H, Sato K, Sekizawa K, Matsuse T, et al. High incidence of aspiration pneumonia in community and hospital-acquired pneumonia in hospitalized patients: a multicenter, prospective study in Japan. J Am Geriatr Soc. 2008;56:577–9.
12. Saitoh E, et al. Survey of distribution of dysphasia patients using Dysphagia Severity Scale 2012 Grant-in-aid of Geriatric Health promotion project, Report of achievement in investigation research of swallowing disorders.
13. Sugiyama M, Takada K, Shinde M, Matsumoto N, Tanaka K, Kiriya Y, et al. National survey of the prevalence of swallowing difficulty and tube feeding use as well as implementation of swallowing evaluation in long-term care settings in Japan. Geriatr Gerontol Int. 2014;14(3):577–81.
14. Saitoh E, Matsuo K, Inamoto Y, Ishikawa M, Tsubahara A. Twenty years of trans-disciplinary approach development for dysphagia rehabilitation in Japan. Dysphagia. 2015;30(1):102–3.

Toyoake, Aichi, Japan Eiichi Saitoh
Toyoake, Aichi, Japan Kannit Pongpipatpaiboon
Toyoake, Aichi, Japan Yoko Inamoto
Toyoake, Aichi, Japan Hitoshi Kagaya

Acknowledgments

This book would not be possible without the gracious support, unfaltering patience, and shared expertise of our coauthors and all the members of the Fujita Swallowing Team. We are fortunate to have a strong transdisciplinary team approach for dysphagia rehabilitation, and we believe our team provides an excellent model for the management of dysphagic patients. We would like to express our deep appreciation and sincerest thanks to Professor Jeffrey B. Palmer, our mentor, for his significant contributions, to Dr. Rachel Mulheren for editorial assistance, and to Dr. Cathy Lazarus for providing patient instruction on how to perform the Effortful swallow. And we must thank our patients, who generously participated in some of the imaging studies presented in this text.

Contents

About the Editors

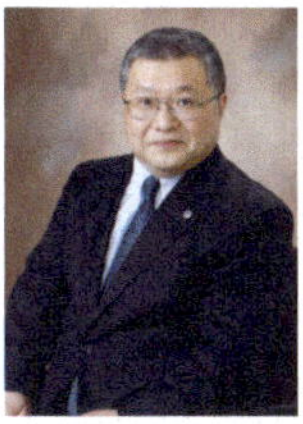

Eiichi Saitoh, MD, DMSc
Physiatrist, Executive Vice President of Fujita Health University, Professor and Chairperson of Department of Rehabilitation Medicine I, School of Medicine, Fujita Health University, Toyoake, Aichi, Japan

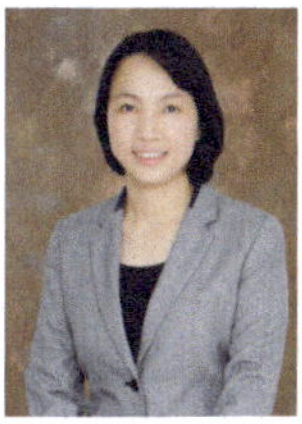

Kannit Pongpipatpaiboon, MD
Physiatrist, Research Fellow of Department of Rehabilitation Medicine I, School of Medicine, Fujita, Health University, Toyoake, Aichi, Japan

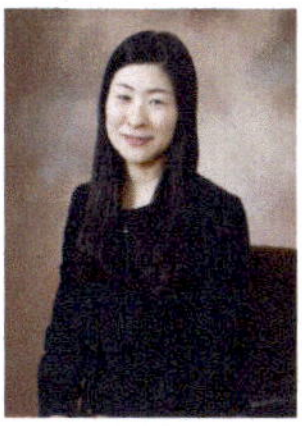

Yoko Inamoto, SLHT, PhD
Speech-Language-Hearing Therapist, Associate Professor of Faculty of Rehabilitation, School of Health Sciences, Fujita Health University, Toyoake, Aichi, Japan

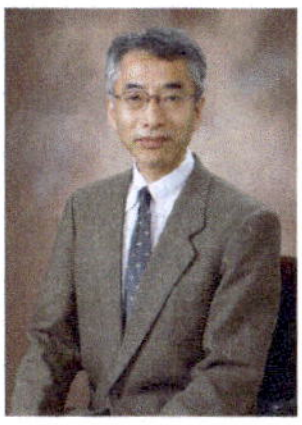

Hitoshi Kagaya, MD, DMSc
Physiatrist, Professor of Department of Rehabilitation Medicine I, School of Medicine, Fujita Health University, Toyoake, Aichi, Japan

About the Authors

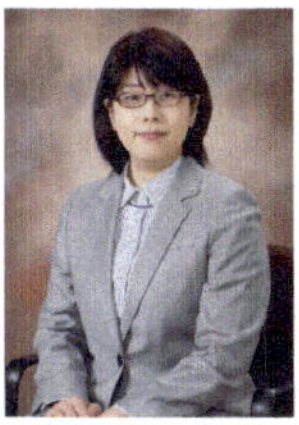

Seiko Shibata, MD, DMSc
Physiatrist, Senior Assistant Professor of Department of Rehabilitation Medicine, School of Medicine, Fujita Health University, Toyoake, Aichi, Japan

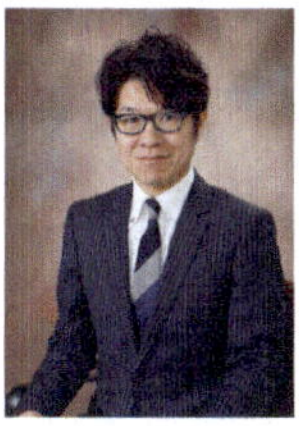

Yoichiro Aoyagi, MD, PhD
Physiatrist, Associate Professor of Department of Rehabilitation Medicine I, School of Medicine, Fujita Health University, Toyoake, Aichi, Japan

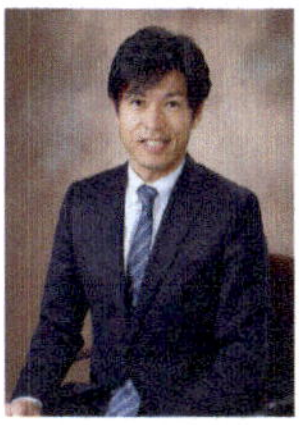

Koichiro Matsuo, DDS, PhD
Dentist, Professor and Chairperson of Department of Dentistry, School of Medicine, Fujita Health University, Toyoake, Aichi, Japan

Abbreviations

3D	Three-dimensional
320-ADCT	320-row area detector CT
ADL	Activities of daily living
CT	Computed tomography
DSS	Dysphagia Severity Scale
EMST	Expiratory muscle-strengthening exercise
ESS	Eating Status Scale
FHUR	Fujita Health University Rehabilitation Complex
FIM	Functional independence measure
HRM	High-resolution manometry
JSDR	Japan Society of Dysphagia Rehabilitation
LES	Lower esophageal sphincter
MEP	Maximum expiratory pressure
mGy	Milligray
MPR	Multiplanar reconstruction
mSv	Millisievert
MWST	Modified water swallowing test
NG	Nasogastric tube
RSST	Repetitive saliva swallowing test
SLHT	Speech-language-hearing pathologist
SWR	Swallowing ward rounds
Threshold PEP™	Threshold positive expiratory pressure device
TOR-BSST©	Toronto Bedside Swallowing Screening Test
TVFs	True vocal folds
UES	Upper esophageal sphincter
VE	Videoendoscopy
VF	Videofluorography
WST	Water swallowing test
W/V	Weight/Volume

Part I
Overview and Physiology

Chapter 1
Overview of Structures and Essential Terms

Kannit Pongpipatpaiboon, Yoko Inamoto, Koichiro Matsuo, Yoichiro Aoyagi, Seiko Shibata, and Hitoshi Kagaya

Abstract This chapter discusses common dysphagia terminology. A common understanding of important terms relevant to dysphagia enables healthcare professionals to communicate clearly and rapidly. The basic knowledge of anatomical structures associated with swallowing is fundamental to understanding the whole swallow process including the evaluation and treatment of dysphagia.

1.1 Terminology of Dysphagia

Swallowing is one of the most frequent activities of humans. Swallowing serves as a vital primary function to ensure nutrition and hydration and contributes to quality of life. Specific terminology is used among healthcare workers to communicate in a common language and is used every day for speaking and writing in medical charts.

A description of the common terms used in the field of dysphagia is provided in Table 1.1.

K. Pongpipatpaiboon • Y. Aoyagi • S. Shibata • H. Kagaya
Department of Rehabilitation Medicine I, School of Medicine, Fujita Health University, Toyoake, Aichi, Japan
e-mail: ning665@gmail.com; yyy@rc5.so-net.ne.jp; sshibata@fujita-hu.ac.jp; hkagaya2@fujita-hu.ac.jp

Y. Inamoto (✉)
Faculty of Rehabilitation, School of Health Sciences, Fujita Health University, Toyoake, Aichi, Japan
e-mail: inamoto@fujita-hu.ac.jp

K. Matsuo
Department of Dentistry, School of Medicine, Fujita Health University, Toyoake, Aichi, Japan
e-mail: kmatsuo@fujita-hu.ac.jp

E. Saitoh et al. (eds.), *Dysphagia Evaluation and Treatment*,
https://doi.org/10.1007/978-981-10-5032-9_1

Table 1.1 Terminology of dysphagia[a]

Swallowing/deglutition	A series of movements that promote bolus transportation from the mouth to the stomach
Eating/ingestion	The process of taking a bolus into the body by mouth
Eating disorder	A psychological disorder characterized by abnormal or disturbed eating behaviors (e.g., anorexia nervosa, bulimia nervosa)
Dys-	Impaired or abnormal
Phag-	Eating
Eating problem/dysphagia	Eating failure or dysfunction, defined as a disturbance of the passage of a swallowed bolus from the mouth to the stomach
Aspiration	Entry of saliva, liquid, or food into the airway under the level of the true vocal folds
Penetration	Entry of swallowed material into the laryngeal vestibule during swallowing, as above of the level of the true vocal folds
Retention	Presence of a residual swallowed bolus locating in the oral cavity, vallecula, and/or hypopharynx (pyriform sinus) that is left behind after the swallow

[a]Additional terminology is shown in Appendix (Table 1.2)

1.2 Overview of Structures

Fundamental knowledge of the anatomy and motor control of eating and swallowing is imperative and serves as an important basis for evaluating the physiology of the swallow. Swallowing is a complicated sequence of movements. A normal swallow requires the precise coordination of more than 30 muscles located within and around the oral cavity, pharynx, larynx, and esophagus. These muscles are controlled by cranial and peripheral nerves that are centrally mediated via the brain stem (mainly the medulla oblongata as the swallowing center) and cooperate with the cortical and subcortical regions of the brain [1, 2].

1.2.1 Anatomical Structures [1–3]

The oral cavity serves as the entrance to both the digestive pathway and upper airway. The tongue rests on the floor on the mouth, exposing both the oral and pharyngeal surfaces. The arched opening of the posterior oral cavity is bordered by the fauces, which separate the oral cavity from the pharynx. The pharyngeal wall consists of three main pharyngeal constrictor muscle groups (the superior, middle, and inferior parts) and long pharyngeal muscles (stylopharyngeus, salpingopharyngeus, and palatopharyngeus). The upper esophageal sphincter (UES) is defined as a high-pressure zone located at the pharyngoesophageal junction and has a semicircular shape in the horizontal view. It consists of three muscular portions: the inferior fibers of the inferior pharyngeal constrictor, the cricopharyngeal muscle, and the upper fibers of the esophagus. The UES contracts at rest and relaxes during swallowing to allow a swallowed bolus to enter the esophagus and to prevent regurgitation of bolus from esophagus and stomach (Figs. 1.1 and 1.2).

The hyoid bone plays an important role in swallowing function. The suprahyoid muscles, which include the mylohyoid, geniohyoid, anterior and posterior bellies of the digastric, and stylohyoid, and one of the infrahyoid muscles, thyrohyoid, play one of the key roles in opening of the UES because they control hyoid and laryngeal excursion in the superoanterior direction, allowing a bolus to pass into the esophagus. The larynx acts as an airway valve, separating the trachea from the upper aerodigestive tract. The airway is protected by laryngeal closure, a process that occurs at three levels: approximation of the true vocal folds (TVFs, glottis), approximation of the false vocal folds, and approximation of the aryepiglottic folds to the base of the epiglottis. The tongue base, pharynx, epiglottis, larynx, and UES comprise the oropharynx and hypopharynx. Three pockets or recesses exist in the oropharyngeal area (vallecula) and in the hypopharyngeal area (two pyriform sinuses), providing a physiologic storage area for food and fluid and decreasing the risk of aspiration. Figure 1.1 provides an overall image of the anatomical structures in the oral cavity, pharynx, and larynx. The swallowing muscles that contribute to the pharyngeal stage are illustrated in Appendix (Figs. 1.4 and 1.5).

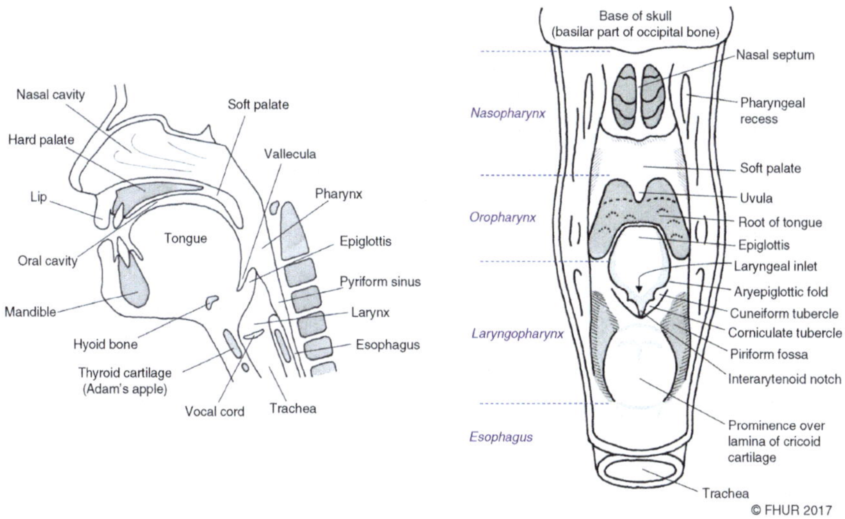

Fig. 1.1 Illustration of the anatomical structures (including oral cavity, pharynx, and larynx) contributing to the swallowing function

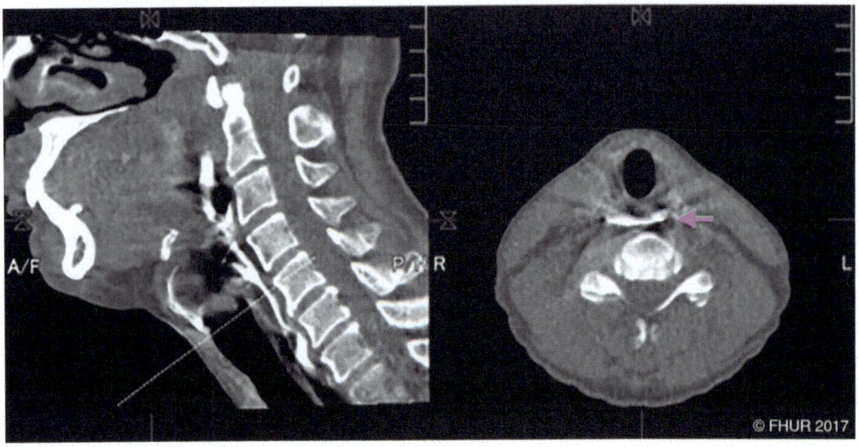

Fig. 1.2 Two-plane computed tomography images of the upper esophageal sphincter illustrate its semicircular shape in the horizontal view at the pharyngoesophageal junction

Fig. 1.3 Diagram of neural control of the pharyngeal stage of swallowing. *NTS* nucleus tractus solitaries; *BS-SW* brain stem swallowing center; *CPG* central pattern generator; *VLM* ventrolateral medulla; *NA* nucleus ambiguous

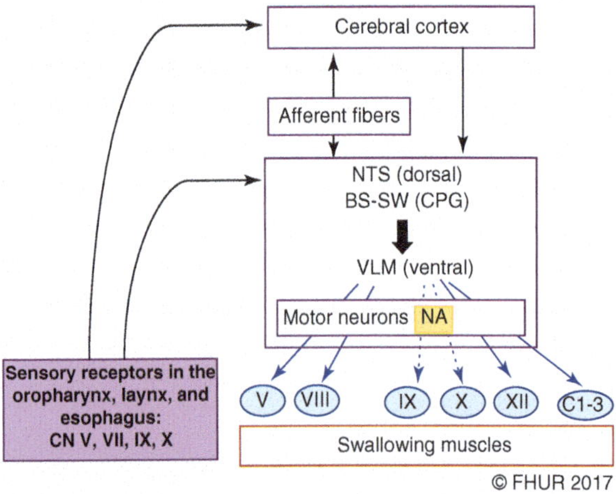

1.2.2 Neural Control of Swallowing [1, 4]

Swallowing is a dynamic process involving complex neuronal networks with volitional and reflexive components. The parts of the central nervous system that control swallowing are mainly the supratentorium (cortical and subcortical cortex) and infratentorium (brain stem). These central networks collaborate with the peripheral nervous system, including several cranial nerves that control sensorimotor swallowing function, to integrate coordination of several structures and muscles as illustrated in Fig. 1.3 and Appendix (Table 1.3).

Appendix

Additional Terminology of Dysphagia

Table 1.2 Additional terminology of dysphagia

Drooling	Defined as flowing of food, liquid, or saliva outside of the mouth unintentionally
Nasal regurgitation	Passing out of food from the oral cavity into the nasal cavity
Pharyngeal regurgitation	Swallowed bolus flows back into the pharynx through the junction of pharynx and esophagus passing the cricopharyngeal sphincter
Gastroesophageal regurgitation	Retrograde movement of the stomach's contents back up into the esophagus

Swallowing Muscles Contributing to the Pharyngeal Stage

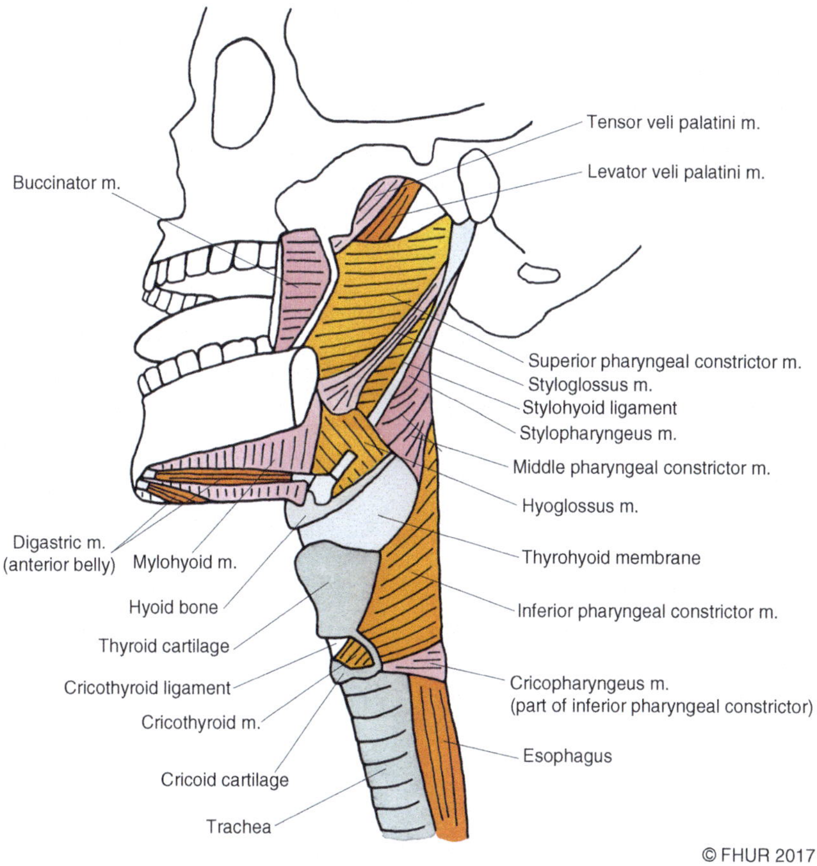

Fig. 1.4 Lateral view of the pharynx illustrating constrictor and suspensory muscles of the pharynx as viewed from the side (*m* muscle)

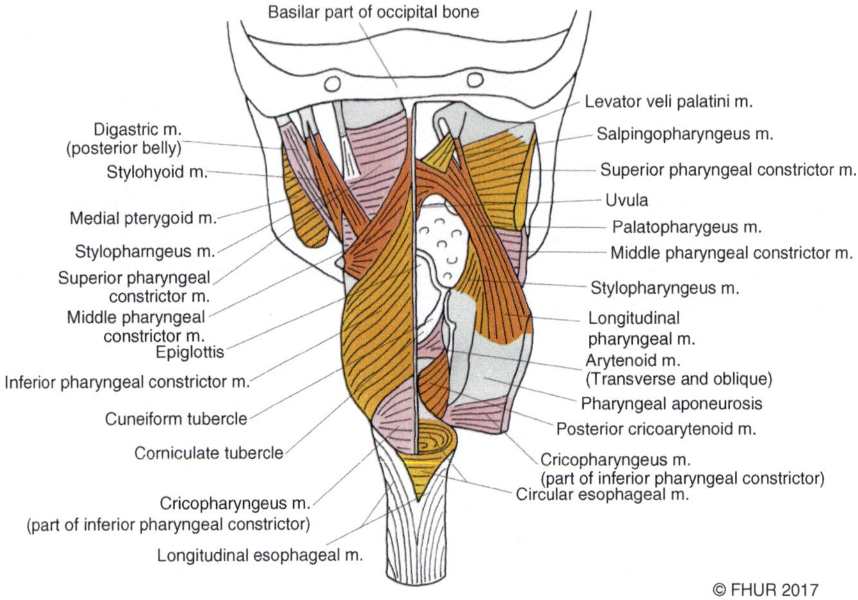

Fig. 1.5 Pharyngeal muscles seen in the posterior view and with the right side of the pharynx cut open, allowing it to be viewed from the inside (*m* muscle)

Neural Control of Swallowing

Table 1.3 Major swallowing-related muscles, innervations, and actions

Category	Muscle	Innervation	Action
Base of tongue	Hyoglossus	XII	Retraction of base of tongue
	Styloglossus		
	Palatoglossus	X	
Pharyngeal constrictors	Superior pharyngeal constrictor	X	Generating positive pressure to the bolus tail through superiorly to inferiorly sequential contractions
	Middle pharyngeal constrictor		
UES	Thyropharyngeus		
	Cricopharyngeus		Contracting tonically at rest and relaxing during swallowing
Long pharyngeus	Stylopharyngeus	X	Pharyngeal shortening, assisting laryngeal elevation
	Salpingopharyngeus	X	
	Palatopharyngeus	X	

Table 1.3 (continued)

Category	Muscle	Innervation	Action
Suprahyoid	Geniohyoid	C1	Hyolaryngeal superoanterior movement of trajectory
	Mylohyoid	V	
	Digastrics	V	
	Stylohyoid	VII	
Infrahyoid	Thyrohyoid	XII, C1	Depressing and posteriorly displacing hyoid and larynx
	Sternohyoid	C1–C3	
	Sternothyroid		
	Omohyoid		

References

1. Shaw SM, Martino R. The normal swallow: muscular and neurophysiological control. Otolaryngol Clin N Am. 2013;46(6):937–56. doi:10.1016/j.otc.2013.09.006.
2. Matsuo K, Palmer JB. Anatomy and physiology of feeding and swallowing: normal and abnormal. Phys Med Rehabil Clin N Am. 2008;19(4):691–707.
3. Logemann JA. Evaluation and treatment of swallowing disorders. 2nd ed. Austin, TX: Pro-Ed; 1998.
4. Malandraki G, Robbins J. Dysphagia. In: Barnes MP, Good DC, editors. Handbook of clinical neurology, vol. 110. New York: Elsevier; 2013. p. 255–71.

Chapter 2
Evolution and Development of Human Swallowing

Kannit Pongpipatpaiboon, Yoko Inamoto, Koichiro Matsuo, Yoichiro Aoyagi, Seiko Shibata, and Hitoshi Kagaya

Abstract This chapter will describe the human swallowing in comparison with other mammals.

Besides, the context will focus on swallowing and feeding development in infants. The basic knowledge of how evolutionary and developmental changes of human swallowing allows an insight into which swallowing-related problems may directly relate.

An understanding of the evolution of human swallowing begins from a comparative mammalian context. The larynx is a focal point in this comparison. Many other mammals, such as the rat, horse, pig, cat, and others, have remarkably similar anatomical templates of the structures involved in swallowing (Fig. 2.1).

The position of the larynx is relatively high in the neck relative to the base of the cranium. The larynx is located in the opening of the intranarial array, providing a continuous airway from the nose to the lungs. Other than the anatomically high position of the larynx in many other mamals, the part of the epiglottis that touches or overlaps above the soft palate (so-called intranarial larynx) permits the margins of the soft palate to seal the airway from food passage. This structure enables the larynx to open directly into the nasopharynx and generates a physical separation of the two pathways (breathing and swallowing) to ensure survival. Furthermore, the

K. Pongpipatpaiboon • Y. Aoyagi • S. Shibata • H. Kagaya
Department of Rehabilitation Medicine I, School of Medicine, Fujita Health University, Toyoake, Aichi, Japan
e-mail: ning665@gmail.com; yyy@rc5.so-net.ne.jp; sshibata@fujita-hu.ac.jp; hkagaya2@fujita-hu.ac.jp

Y. Inamoto (✉)
Faculty of Rehabilitation, School of Health Sciences, Fujita Health University, Toyoake, Aichi, Japan
e-mail: inamoto@fujita-hu.ac.jp

K. Matsuo
Department of Dentistry, School of Medicine, Fujita Health University, Toyoake, Aichi, Japan
e-mail: kmatsuo@fujita-hu.ac.jp

E. Saitoh et al. (eds.), *Dysphagia Evaluation and Treatment*,
https://doi.org/10.1007/978-981-10-5032-9_2

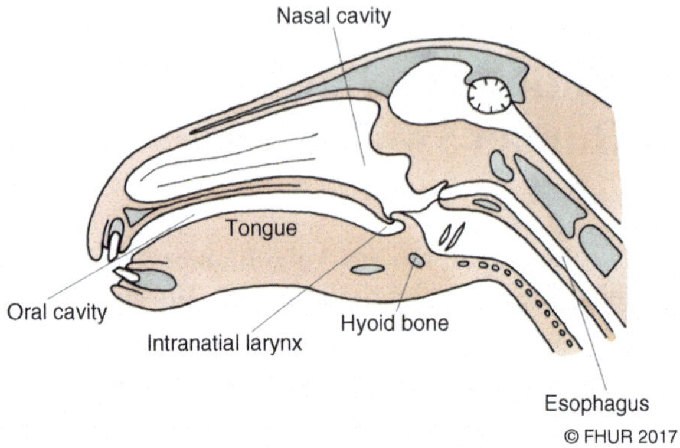

Fig. 2.1 Illustration of the midsagittal section of the head and neck regions of the horse

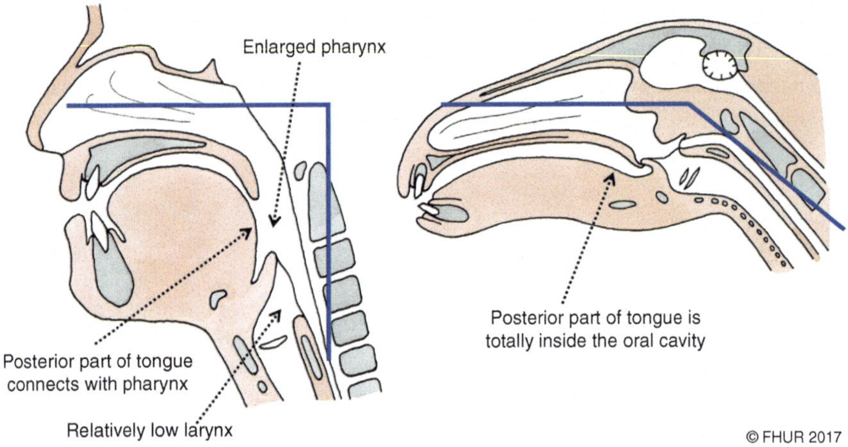

Fig. 2.2 Comparative oropharyngolaryngeal structures between humans and other mammals

tongue in other mammals lies almost entirely within the oral cavity; no portion is present in the pharyngeal part [1, 2].

Comparison of the oropharyngolaryngeal anatomy in humans and other mammals (Fig. 2.2) illustrates three main principles of swallowing:

1. In the standing position, the oral and pharyngeal regions in humans are at a right angle to each other, bending sharply at 90°, as shown in Fig. 2.2. In contrast, the angle between the oral and pharyngeal regions is relatively flat in other mammals. This means that in humans, liquid easily enters the larynx before flowing into the esophagus.
2. The pharynx of other mammals is comparatively small, with the laryngeal opening to the nasal cavity (intranarial larynx). This structure therefore serves as a protective mechanism to prevent aspiration during swallowing.
3. The entire posterior part of other mammals' tongues is located inside the mouth. In contrast, the posterior part of the human's tongue is connected to the pharynx, forming part of the anterior pharyngeal wall (Fig. 2.3).

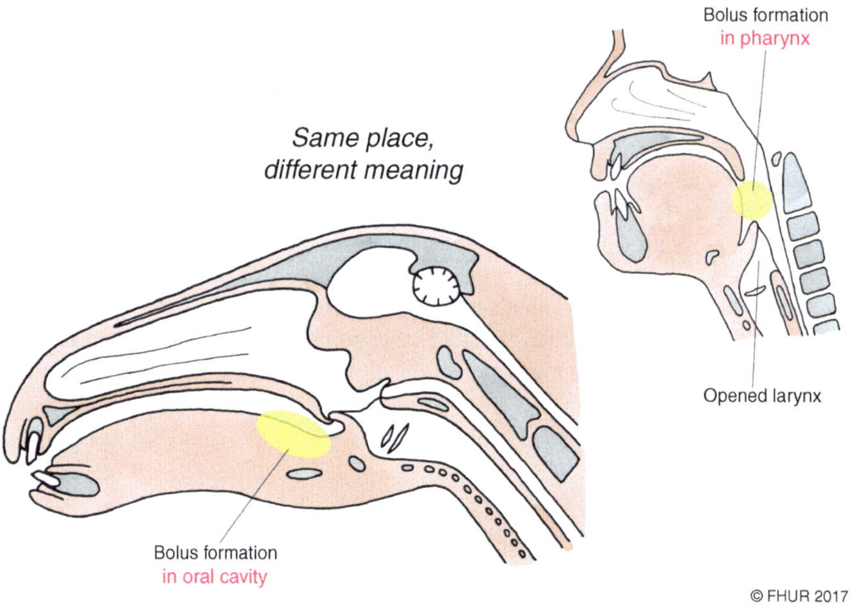

Fig. 2.3 Comparison of the location of bolus formation in humans and other mammals. Although the bolus is located at the same place (posterior part of the tongue), the significance in terms of swallowing differs. Bolus formation occurs in the oral cavity in other mammals and in part of the pharynx in humans. This is because in humans, the posterior part of the tongue is opened in larynx. Thus, the bolus cannot stay here during chewing

These structural differences arose from the evolutional demand for rich phonation in the human being. Thus, the pathways of breathing and swallowing converged in the pharynx, and the functions of this common pathway have no clear separation in humans. This results in a higher risk of aspirating food from the shared oropharynx into the larynx. Although this anatomical arrangement enables safe swallowing in other mammals, it significantly limits the array of sounds (phonation). This limitation in the range of sounds that can be produced is similar to that in a human infant.

2.1 Development of Swallowing in Humans

Proper development of the anatomical structures involved in swallowing is crucial to subsequent normal swallowing function. For this reason, an understanding of the evolution of the normal anatomy involved in the human swallowing mechanism is required. There is clear evidence of differences in the anatomy of the head and neck between infants and adults, and these anatomical differences influence feeding and swallowing [3–5].

The oral cavity in the newborn is totally occupied by the tongue because of the small and slightly retracted lower jaw. The hard palate is flat and no teeth have emerged. Additionally, thicker fat pads are present in the cheeks and provide stability during suckling. Because of these structures, the space in the oral cavity is smaller in newborns than in adults, and infants are more efficient at suckling than chewing. The pharynx is relatively short, and the hyoid bone and larynx lie at a much higher level and closer to the base of the epiglottis than in the adult, providing added airway protection. In addition, the tip of the epiglottis contacts the soft palate at the second cervical level; thus, the larynx opens directly to the nasal cavity, similar to nonhuman mammals as described previously (Fig. 2.4).

These anatomical differences create a separation between the respiratory and digestive routes, affording natural protection of the airway and providing an optimal arrangement for safe feeding.

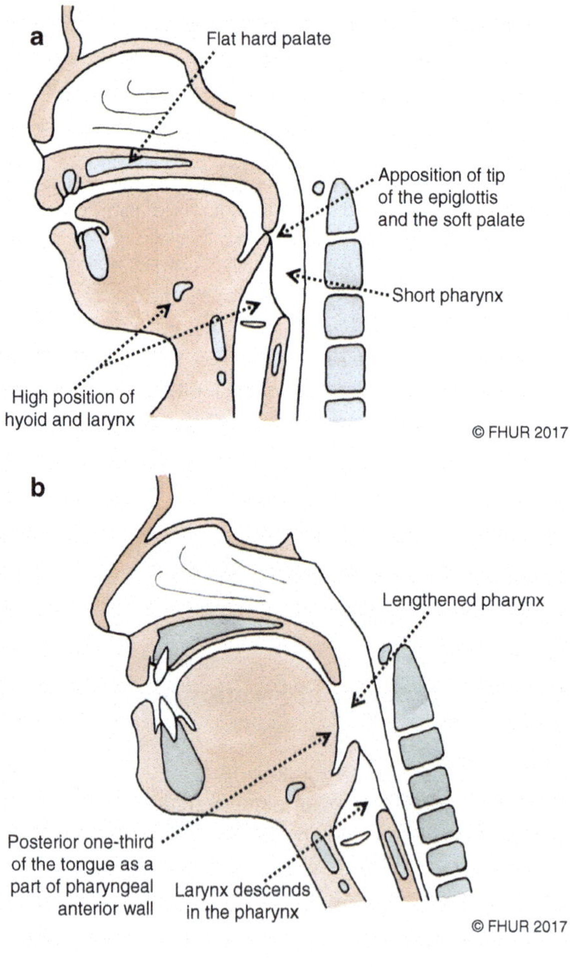

Fig. 2.4 Mouth and pharynx, (**a**) newborn, (**b**) adult in sagittal section

The anatomy involved in swallowing gradually changes as follows throughout development:

- The dentition develops.
- The oral cavity enlarges.
- The larynx descends in the pharynx.
- The pharynx lengthens vertically.
- The posterior one-third of the tongue descends into the pharynx and bends at a right angle relative to the oral portion, lying in a vertical plane and forming the upper anterior wall of the pharynx. The oral cavity and oropharynx are thus open to the nasopharynx and hypopharynx.

The upper aerodigestive tract begins to closely resemble that of an adult by approximately 5 months of age.

This change in the human requires elaboration of airway protection, functionally separating the two pathways. The respiratory and digestive tracts now cross each other in the pharyngeal area, minimizing aspiration protection. This is one reason why older individuals are at higher risk of swallowing problems. Although humans have acquired the disadvantage of pharyngeal swallowing because of anatomical changes, the descent of the larynx provides an advantage. The longer pharyngeal portion enables rich sound production at the vocal folds (phonation) and the ability to fully articulate speech.

References

1. Laitman JT, Reidenberg JS. Specializations of the human upper respiratory and upper digestive systems as seen through comparative and developmental anatomy. Dysphagia. 1993;8:318–25.
2. German RZ, Crompton AW, Thexton AJ. The coordination and interaction between respiration and deglutition in young pigs. J Comp Physiol A. 1998;182:539–47.
3. Logemann JA. Evaluation and treatment of swallowing disorders. 2nd ed. Austin: Pro-Ed; 1998.
4. Delaney AL, Arvedson JC. Development of swallowing and feeding: prenatal through first year of life. Dev Disabil Res Rev. 2008;14(2):105–17.
5. Tutor JD, Gosa MM. Dysphagia and aspiration in children. Pediatr Pulmonol. 2012;47(4):321–37.

Chapter 3
Physiological Models of Swallowing

Kannit Pongpipatpaiboon, Yoko Inamoto, Koichiro Matsuo, Yoichiro Aoyagi, Seiko Shibata, and Hitoshi Kagaya

Abstract Swallowing is a complex activity in humans that involves coordinated activity of the mouth, pharynx, larynx, and esophagus. Thorough knowledge of these physiological processes is necessary to understand the complexity of swallowing and serves as an essential module for explaining the fundamental mechanisms that operate in swallowing activity. In addition, an understanding of the mechanism of swallowing allows us to formulate new questions that serve as the basis for experiments and detect specific problems that must be managed in the clinical setting. The swallowing sequence is divided into stages, each involving different food management behaviors. Two common models of drinking and eating are widely used.

The first is the four-stage sequence model for drinking, and the second is the process model for eating (chew–swallow complex) solid food. In addition to these, a two-stage model comprising the pharyngeal and esophageal stages was recently reported. This model revealed that the isolated pharyngeal swallow, in which the food bolus is not transported by the tongue in the oral cavity, is a part of normal human feeding (Fig. 3.1).

A brief summary of the current understanding of these swallow stages and the differences among them is clearly outlined in the following text.

K. Pongpipatpaiboon • Y. Aoyagi • S. Shibata • H. Kagaya
Department of Rehabilitation Medicine I, School of Medicine, Fujita Health University, Toyoake, Aichi, Japan
e-mail: ning665@gmail.com; yyy@rc5.so-net.ne.jp; sshibata@fujita-hu.ac.jp; hkagaya2@fujita-hu.ac.jp

Y. Inamoto (✉)
Faculty of Rehabilitation, School of Health Sciences, Fujita Health University, Toyoake, Aichi, Japan
e-mail: inamoto@fujita-hu.ac.jp

K. Matsuo
Department of Dentistry, School of Medicine, Fujita Health University, Toyoake, Aichi, Japan
e-mail: kmatsuo@fujita-hu.ac.jp

E. Saitoh et al. (eds.), *Dysphagia Evaluation and Treatment*,
https://doi.org/10.1007/978-981-10-5032-9_3

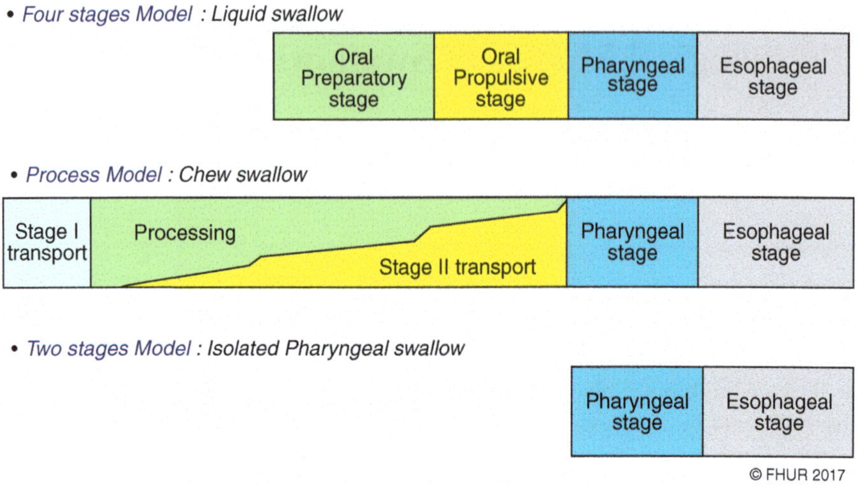

Fig. 3.1 Illustration of three physiological models of swallowing: two-stage, four-stage, and process models

Swallowing is traditionally divided into four stages: the oral preparatory, oral propulsive, pharyngeal, and esophageal stages. The four-stage swallowing model is used to explain the command swallow (swallowing under order during an experiment) and the discrete swallow (one spontaneous swallow) of liquids and the concept that bolus propulsion to the pharynx normally does not occur until the initiation of swallow onset. However, this model does not adequately represent the mechanism of eating and swallowing solid food. One of the most important fundamental differences between the processes of drinking liquids and eating solids, other than the consistency of the food, is the chewing process before swallowing as well as the coordination between chewing and intraoral food transport with swallowing. This means that the major difference is in the oral stage, whereas the pharyngeal and esophageal stages have minor differences (Fig. 3.1).

3.1 Four-Stage Model

The four-stage model comprises the oral preparatory stage, oral propulsive stage, pharyngeal stage, and esophageal stage [1].

3.1.1 Oral Preparatory Stage

A liquid bolus is collected in the anterior part of the oral cavity and placed in a swallow-ready position. Two regions in the oral cavity may hold a liquid bolus prior to initiating the swallow: the floor of the mouth in the anterior part of the oral cavity (dipper type) and the tongue surface against the hard palate (tipper type) [2].

The lips are sealed, and the tongue tip elevates to contact the anterior alveolar ridge and thus prevent drooling. The tongue creates a cuplike shape to entrap the bolus on its dorsum. The posterior part of the oral cavity is closed by tongue–palate contact behind the bolus, which is mainly controlled by the palatoglossus muscle, to prevent premature leakage into the oropharynx before the swallow.

3.1.2 Oral Propulsive Stage

The tip and sides of the tongue are anchored to the alveolar ridge. The posterior region of the tongue is depressed to open the posterior portion of the oral cavity. The bolus is subsequently propelled from the oral cavity to the pharynx through the fauces by a stripping action of the tongue along the palate from the anterior to posterior part using a squeezing mechanism [3]. The bolus is pushed to the back of the mouth and toward the pharynx (Fig. 3.2).

3.1.3 Pharyngeal Stage

The pharyngeal stage usually occurs subsequent to the oral transport stage. The pharyngeal swallow is voluntarily initiated by propelling the bolus from the pharynx into the esophagus. This stage is the most critical stage of the swallow because airway protection occurs, preventing the bolus from entering the respiratory system.

The physiological activities during the pharyngeal stage occur step by step as follows:

1. The soft palate is raised and contacts the lateral and posterior pharyngeal walls primarily by the levator and tensor veli palatini muscles, palatopharyngeus muscle, and superior pharyngeal constrictor muscle, completely closing the velopharyngeal part to isolate the nasopharynx from the oropharynx and prevent food material from entering the nasal cavity (nasal regurgitation).
2. The larynx and hyoid move superiorly and anteriorly by contraction of the suprahyoid and thyrohyoid muscles. This anterosuperior movement of the larynx and hyoid bone is important for several reasons [1, 5, 6]. First, this movement brings the larynx to a position under the tongue base and out of the descending bolus pathway and may facilitate the epiglottis to tilt backward. Second, the elevation

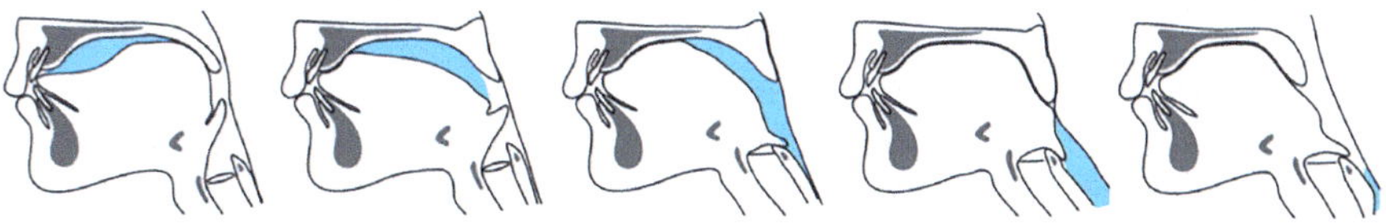

Fig. 3.2 Diagram of normal swallowing of liquid bolus. The bolus is readily held between the anterior surface of the tongue and hard palate. The posterior tongue–palate contact separates the oral cavity and pharynx. The posterior tongue drops down and the soft palate rises with swallowing onset, allowing the bolus to flow into the pharynx (Reproduced from [4] with permission)

of the pharynx and larynx shortens and widens the pharynx, creating a vacuum of negative pressure (suction force) in the hypopharynx to pull the bolus into the esophagus. Third, this action creates a pulling force to open the cricopharyngeal muscle and UES by tracking the cricoid cartilage up and forward away from the posterior pharyngeal wall.

3. The base of the tongue is retracted toward the posterior pharyngeal wall, preventing the food from reentering the mouth and delivering the bolus to the pharynx by the tongue's driving force.
4. The contractions of the pharyngeal constrictor muscles from the upper to lower part help to squeeze the bolus downward, reducing the pharyngeal volume and increasing the pharyngeal pressure.
5. Closure of the larynx occurs. Laryngeal closure involves three main aspects: the TVC, laryngeal vestibule (false vocal folds and aryepiglottic folds), and epiglottic inversion [7–9].

   - TVC: TVC closure has been described as the first event of laryngeal closure [7, 8]. Recent CT study [10], however, revealed that timing of TVC closure was adjusted by the bolus viscosity, suggesting TVC as adaptable component of swallow. TVC closure may occur before swallowing or at any time during swallowing responding to bolus flow.
   - At the level of the laryngeal vestibule, the false vocal folds contract, and the arytenoids tilt forward and inward to contact the epiglottic base.
   - The epiglottis is retroverted. It folds backward over the top of the larynx, and the base of the epiglottis contacts the adducted arytenoids, tilting forward. This mechanism protects the airway, diverting the bolus into the pyriform sinus by sliding down on the epiglottis.

6. The pharyngeal stage ends when the UES relaxes and permits the bolus to enter the esophagus entirely. The opening of the UES is dependent upon the following three conditions [11]: relaxation of the tonically contracted UES; traction forces through the anterior hyolaryngeal excursion; the distensibility property of muscles, which allows the UES to stretch and accommodate the bolus passage; and the increase in intrabolus pressure with the expanding effect of the approaching bolus.

3.1.4 Esophageal Stage [1, 5, 12]

This stage starts once the bolus passes through the UES. The UES is under tension in the resting state and relaxes while food passes into the esophagus. After the bolus has successfully entered the esophagus, the cricopharyngeal muscle returns to its contracted state to prevent the bolus from flowing back into the hypopharynx in a retrograde manner (pharyngeal regurgitation), which can possibly lead to aspiration.

Primary esophageal peristalsis is activated in response to arrival of the bolus; this stretches the esophageal lumen when it occurs in connection with the pharyngeal swallow, propelling the bolus toward the lower esophageal sphincter (LES). The wavelike process of secondary esophageal peristalsis then occurs by local distension to squeeze the bolus into the stomach under control by the autonomic nervous system. Likewise, gravity partly assists bolus transfer in the upright position. The esophageal transit time should normally range from approximately 8 to 20 s [13]. The LES relaxes so that the bolus can enter the stomach. The LES is also contracted at rest, as is the UES, after the bolus passes into the stomach to prevent gastroesophageal regurgitation. The swallowing process is complete at this point, and digestion begins after the bolus enters the stomach through the LES.

3.2 Process Model

The process model is used to describe the mechanism of eating and the chewing process before swallowing solid food [4, 14–17].

3.2.1 Oral Stage

As previously mentioned, it is important to note that highly variable differences are present depending on the food consistency (solid versus liquid) in the oral stage. The process model is used to describe the process of mastication and swallowing of solid food. The solid food is first taken into the mouth and chewed in the oral cavity. The fauces is not sealed because the tongue and soft palate move continuously during mastication and the food bolus moves down into the pharynx prior to swallowing. Thus, pre-swallowing bolus formation of solid foods usually occurs in the oropharynx, whereas pre-swallowing bolus formation of liquids occurs in the mouth.

3.2.2 Stage I Transport

In the process model, after the food has been placed in the mouth, it is moved from the tongue surface to the postcanine region (molar area) by pulling back movement of tongue. The tongue then rotates laterally and places the food on the occlusal surfaces of the lower teeth for food processing in the molar region; this is called the pullback mechanism (Fig. 3.3).

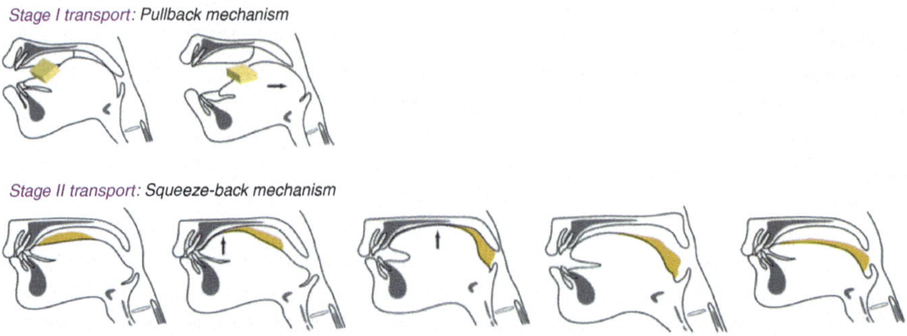

Fig. 3.3 Schematic diagrams of mechanisms involved in stage I and stage II transport. *Pullback mechanism*: The food is carried posteriorly on the tongue surface to the molar region during intraoral transport. *Squeeze-back mechanism*: The food is transported posteriorly by pressing the tongue against the palate (Reproduced from [4] with permission)

3.2.3 Food Processing

Food processing immediately follows stage I transport. The food is continuously chewed in the oral cavity and softened by moistening with saliva until the food bolus reaches optimal cohesiveness and is ready for swallowing (triturated food).

The tongue moves cyclically, anteroposteriorly, mediolaterally, and rotationally during chewing to carry pieces of food from side to side. Additionally, tongue movement in the vertical dimensions coordinates with jaw and hyoid bone movements during this process.

3.2.4 Stage II Transport

Stage II transport is an active process driven by squeezing of the tongue upward against the palate. The swallow-ready chewed solid food is placed on the dorsal surface of the tongue and propelled back from the oral cavity through the fauces to the oropharyngeal tongue surface by the squeeze-back mechanism (Fig. 3.3).

Stage II transport occurs intermittently throughout the motion cycles of the jaw during food processing; accordingly, a portion of chewed solid food commonly reaches the oropharynx (either in the upper oropharynx or vallecula) or the hypopharynx at the time of swallow onset. As seen in Fig. 3.1 (the process model), food processing and stage II transport overlap substantially in time.

Clear evidence shows that stage II transport is primarily actively driven and accomplished by the tongue squeezing food back along the palate; it does not depend on gravity. Chewed food is swallowed and actively transported to the vallecula; however, some liquid within two-phase foods may move into the hypopharynx under the influence of gravity (chew–swallow complex) (Fig. 3.4).

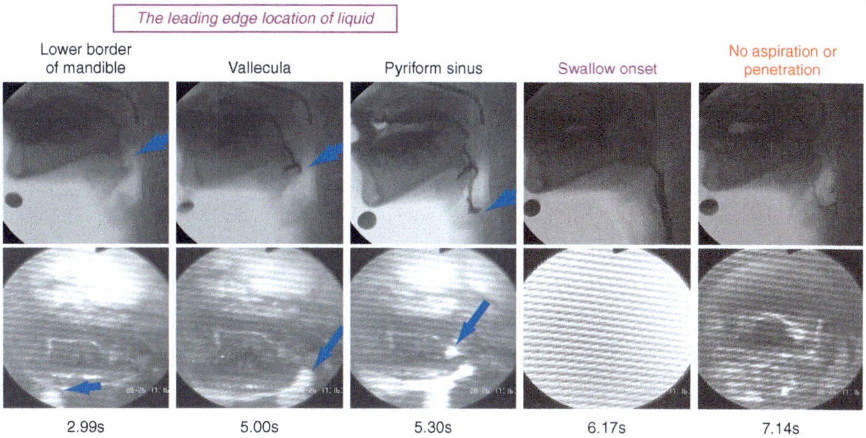

Fig. 3.4 Eating of a two-phase food (corn beef hash and liquid barium) observed simultaneously by videofluorography and videoendoscopy in a healthy subject. Arrows indicate the leading edge of the barium until swallowing (Reproduced from [18] with permission)

The bolus gradually accumulates on the oropharyngeal surface of the tongue and in the vallecula; it may be collected for up to 10 s before the onset of the pharyngeal swallow. This part of the process exhibits individual variability. A person's overall chewing behavior influences the timing of food transport and swallow initiation and must be considered while evaluating swallow disorders. Early bolus arrival in the oropharynx or hypopharynx is associated with a higher risk of aspiration, particularly in individuals with impairments in their swallowing and airway protection mechanisms. Upon completion of bolus aggregation, swallowing is initiated, and the bolus is transported from the pharynx through the UES to the esophagus.

3.3 Two-Stage Model

The pharyngeal stage usually occurs subsequent to the oral transport stage. Nevertheless, the swallow can be initiated at the pharyngeal level during normal human feeding; this is called the isolated pharyngeal swallow, wherein no bolus is transported from the oral cavity [19]. This appears to be similar to the phenomenon observed in an experimental animal model in which the swallow was triggered by direct infusion of water into the pharynx. The reflexive or pharyngeal swallow occurs nonvolitionally in response to pharyngeal stimulation. This phenomenon suggests that the isolated pharyngeal swallow is likely an airway protective mechanism to prevent aspiration.

3.4 Coordination of Deglutition and Respiration

Coordination of respiration and swallowing is vital for airway protection because these two processes share a common pathway that crosses in the pharynx [20, 21]. Both breathing and swallowing are under close neuronal control by a brain stem central pattern generator. Respiration and swallowing have tight temporal coordination. A large amount of evidence shows that swallowing mostly occurs during the expiratory phase. Respiration is inhibited to accommodate swallowing (this is called swallow apnea) due to central inhibition of the brain stem, which has been described as an important mechanism of airway protection. The duration of the respiratory pause that occurs involuntarily during each swallow is approximately 0.5–1.5 s in healthy adults. Expiration resumes afterward. This typical respiration–swallowing pattern ("exhale–swallow–exhale") is a protective mechanism that reduces the probability of inhalation of food material into the airway after swallowing [21]. This pattern occurs in >75% of the swallows of healthy adults. Although most swallows occur during expiration, swallowing can be initiated during a brief interruption of inspiration; aspiration is prevented by laryngeal adduction. This pattern ("inhale–swallow–exhale") occurs in about 20% of swallows. In rare cases, swallowing is followed by inspiratory flow.

Several factors can vary the conditions of the respiration–swallowing coordination pattern. Advanced age has an impact on the coordination between respiration and deglutition. Older adults have been shown to have prolonged swallow apnea to accommodate swallowing and a higher incidence of inspiration both before and after the swallow. This pattern predisposes older adults to aspiration pneumonia. Likewise, swallows that occur during the inspiratory phase of breathing are more frequent in individuals with cerebrovascular disease, Parkinson's disease, chronic obstructive pulmonary disease, or other neurological diseases and may be related to the rising incidence of aspiration pneumonia due to disruption of this protective mechanism pattern.

Variations in the bolus viscosity and volume also influence the swallow-associated respiratory cycle. During the chew–swallow of solid food in stage II transport of the process model, respiration does not stop when the bolus is transported downward into the vallecula and hypopharynx. This can be a causal factor in the higher risk of aspiration. Similar to sequential liquid swallows, which involve longer durations of the transitional stage (as in drinking with a cup or straw), longer sustainment of airway closure is needed and an additional demand on respiratory–swallowing coordination is present because of a significant increase in the resumption of inspiration after swallowing, especially in the elderly and patients with pulmonary or neurological diseases.

References

1. Matsuo K, Palmer JB. Anatomy and physiology of feeding and swallowing: normal and abnormal. Phys Med Rehabil Clin N Am. 2008;19(4):691–707.
2. Dodds WJ, Taylor AJ, Stewart ET, Kern MK, Logemann JA, Cook IJ. Tipper and dipper types of oral swallows. AJR Am J Roentgenol. 1989;153:1197–9.
3. Ramsey GH, Watson JS, Gramiak R, Weinberg SA. Cinefluorographic analysis of the mechanism of swallowing. Radiology. 1955;64(4):498–518.
4. Palmer JB, Rudin NJ, Lara G, Crompton AW. Coordination of mastication and swallowing. Dysphagia. 1992;7(4):187–200.
5. Shaw SM, Martino R. The normal swallow: muscular and neurophysiological control. Otolaryngol Clin N Am. 2013;46:937–56.
6. McConnel FM. Analysis of pressure generation and bolus transit during pharyngeal swallowing. Laryngoscope. 1988;98(1):71–8.
7. Ardran GM, Kemp FH. The protection of the laryngeal airway during swallowing. Br J Radiol. 1952;25:406–16.
8. Ardran GM, Kemp FH. Closure and opening of the larynx during swallowing. Br J Radiol. 1956;29:205–8.
9. Ekberg O. Closure of the laryngeal vestibule during deglutition. Acta Otolaryngol. 1982;93:123–9.
10. Inamoto Y, Saitoh E, Okada S, Kagaya H, Shibata S, Ota K, et al. The effect of bolus viscosity on laryngeal closure in swallowing: kinematic analysis using 320-row area detector CT. Dysphagia. 2013;28(1):33–42.
11. Cook IJ, Dodds WJ, Dantas RO, Massey B, Kern MK, Lang IM, et al. Opening mechanism of the human upper esophageal sphincter. Am J Phys. 1989;257:748–59.
12. Logemann JA. Evaluation and treatment of swallowing disorders. 2nd ed. Austin, TX: Pro-Ed; 1998.
13. Dodds WJ, Hogan W, Reid D, Stewart E, Arndorfer R. A comparison between primary esophageal peristalsis following wet and dry swallows. J Appl Physiol. 1973;35:851–7.
14. Palmer JB. Bolus aggregation in the oropharynx does not depend on gravity. Arch Phys Med Rehabil. 1998;79:691–6.
15. Hiiemae KM, Palmer JB. Food transport and bolus formation during complete feeding sequences on foods of different initial consistency. Dysphagia. 1999;14(1):31–42.
16. Saitoh E, Shibata S, Matsuo K, Baba M, Fujii W, Palmer JB. Chewing and food consistency: effects on bolus transport and swallow initiation. Dysphagia. 2007;22(2):100–7.
17. Palmer JB, Hiiemae KM, Matsuo K, Haishima H. Volitional control of food transport and bolus formation during feeding. Physiol Behav. 2007;91(1):66–70.
18. Saitoh E, Ueda K. Dysphagia rehabilitation. 3rd ed. Tokyo: Ishiyaku; 2016. (Japanese).
19. Kagaya H, Yokoyama M, Saitoh E, Kanamori D, Susa C, German RZ, et al. Isolated pharyngeal swallow exists during normal human feeding. Tohoku J Exp Med. 2015;236(1):39–43.
20. Matsuo K, Hiiemae KM, Gonzalez-Fernandez M, Palmer JB. Respiration during feeding on solid food: alterations in breathing during mastication, pharyngeal bolus aggregation, and swallowing. J Appl Physiol. 2008;104:674–81.
21. Matsuo K, Palmer JB. Coordination of mastication, swallowing and breathing. Jpn Dent Sci Rev. 2009;45(1):31–40.

Part II
Clinical Approaches

Chapter 4
Dysphagia from the Viewpoint of Rehabilitation Medicine

Kannit Pongpipatpaiboon, Yoko Inamoto, Yoichiro Aoyagi, Seiko Shibata, Hitoshi Kagaya, and Koichiro Matsuo

Abstract Dysphagia is a common problem in medical situations. Many disease processes are associated with a high incidence of dysphagia. Individuals with dysphagia may have multiple problems and need assessment and treatment that requires the input of multiple health professional specialists. Good team approach will increase the efficacy of dysphagia treatment.

Dysphagia is also common in aging societies because of the physical changes in structure and function that occur in these populations [1–5]. However, swallowing disorders have various etiologies and can affect persons of any age.

As mentioned in the first section, the oropharyngolaryngeal space is involved in multiple functions including breathing, phonation, and swallowing. These three functions exhibit trade-off relationships. Accordingly, this space is associated with a risk of choking during swallowing, and any dysfunction in this system can lead to dysphagia and possible aspiration. Dysphagia adversely affects the patient's eating ability, which is one of the great pleasures in life. Some patients face long-standing swallowing problems with adverse consequences [4–9] such as malnutrition, dehydration, aspiration pneumonia, and asphyxiation, significantly reducing their quality of life as well as increasing their rehabilitation time, need for care provision, and

K. Pongpipatpaiboon • Y. Aoyagi • S. Shibata • H. Kagaya
Department of Rehabilitation Medicine I, School of Medicine,
Fujita Health University, Toyoake, Aichi, Japan
e-mail: ning665@gmail.com; yyy@rc5.so-net.ne.jp;
sshibata@fujita-hu.ac.jp; hkagaya2@fujita-hu.ac.jp

Y. Inamoto (✉)
Faculty of Rehabilitation, School of Health Sciences, Fujita Health University,
Toyoake, Aichi, Japan
e-mail: inamoto@fujita-hu.ac.jp

K. Matsuo
Department of Dentistry, School of Medicine, Fujita Health University, Toyoake, Aichi, Japan
e-mail: kmatsuo@fujita-hu.ac.jp

E. Saitoh et al. (eds.), *Dysphagia Evaluation and Treatment*,
https://doi.org/10.1007/978-981-10-5032-9_4

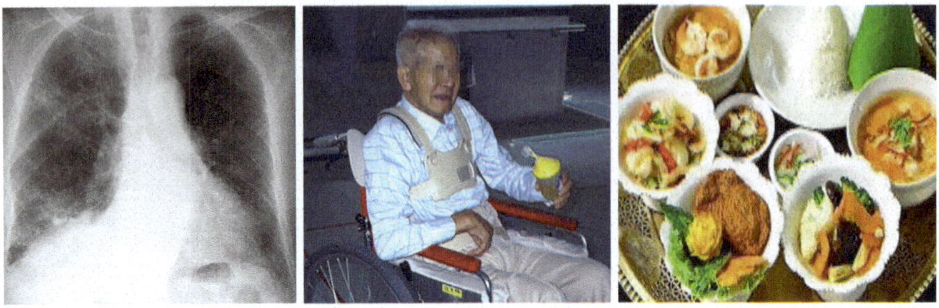

Fig. 4.1 Serious problems in dysphagic patients from the viewpoint of rehabilitation medicine

need for long-term care assistance [10–12] (Fig. 4.1). Thus, the consequences of dysphagia include significant morbidity and mortality and increased healthcare costs. A well-coordinated care plan can prevent or minimize the development of dysphagia-related complications.

It is imperative that both specialists and general physicians recognize and understand the contribution of dysphagia to patients with various conditions and develop the ability to prioritize proper evaluation and treatment plans. There is a definite need to increase the importance of dedicated patient care and research in the emerging field of dysphagia.

Treatment of dysphagia has been a new task in rehabilitation medicine during the past few decades. Japanese insurance began coverage of dysphagia treatment in 1994. One year later, the The Japanese Society of Dysphagia Rehabilitation (JSDR) was established. The JSDR had 1,600 members in 1996 and has rapidly expanded its membership since. The objective of this unique society is to perform activities related to research, education, dissemination, and structuralization in the field of dysphagia rehabilitation to resolve problems in individuals with eating and swallowing difficulties.

Annual publication of the *Japanese Journal of Dysphagia Rehabilitation* began in 1997. The field of dysphagia rehabilitation began growing thereafter and has progressed more rapidly since 2000. The JSDR also holds annual meetings to promote the progress and spread of knowledge regarding the diagnosis of, evaluation of, and transdisciplinary approaches to dysphagia through presentation of papers and their practical applications, exchange of knowledge and welfare activities, encouragement of continuing medical education for members, and enhancement of mutual coordination and cooperation among members and related domestic and foreign societies.

As shown in Fig. 4.2, dysphagia rehabilitation in Japan started with the clinical application of videofluorography (VF) in the mid-1980s. The first original paper to mention the usefulness of VF for rehabilitative approach was published in 1986. This paper described analysis of the postural effect on dysphagia management.

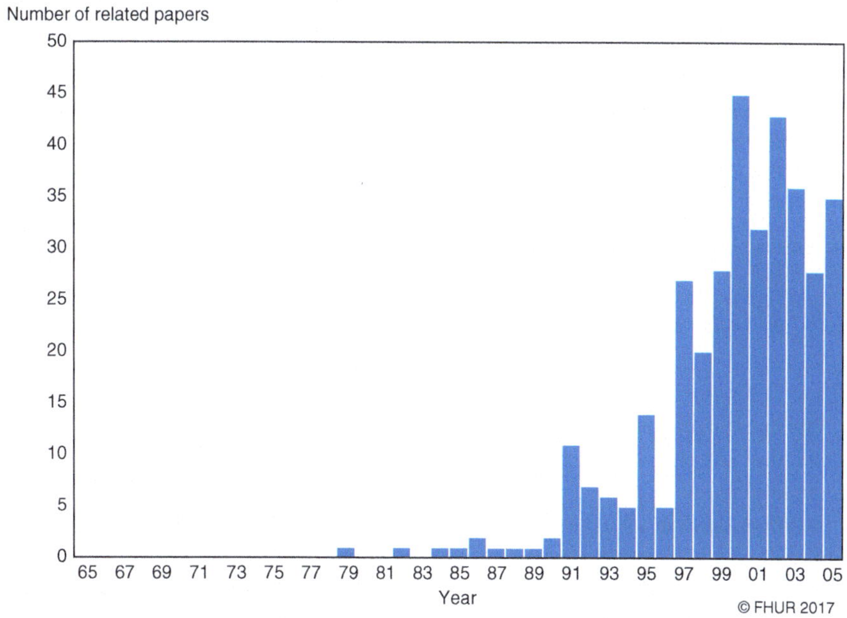

Fig. 4.2 Bar chart showing the number of articles related to dysphagia in four major rehabilitation journals in Japan (Jpn J Rehab Med since 1965, Sogo Rehab since 1973, J Clin Rehab since 1992, and Jpn J Dysphagia Rehab since 1997)

4.1 Dysphagia Team Development in Japan

The concept of a team approach to swallowing disorders has developed over time [13–15]. The team approach is generally divided into the following three categories according to the relationships among disciplines: the multidisciplinary approach, interdisciplinary approach, and transdisciplinary approach (Table 4.1).

The transdisciplinary teamwork model is suitable for dysphagia rehabilitation and is common in Japan, especially for the small facilities that may face shortages in the number and kinds of healthcare workers [16, 17]. In this model, participating disciplines complement the scope of one another without rigid borders between them. Practitioners from various disciplines freely share fundamental knowledge, perspectives, and skills. This model thus leads to more efficient integration, permits better understanding, and achieves more effective evaluation. The JSDR was founded under the concept of a transdisciplinary team approach for dysphagia rehabilitation.

The swallowing team at the FHUR provides one of the best examples of the attitude that a transdisciplinary team should exhibit. This team comprises professionals in several fields: physiatrists, dentists, certified dysphagia nurses, speech-language-hearing therapists (SLHTs), otolaryngologists, dental hygienists, dieticians, and ward nurses.

Table 4.1 Team healthcare approach to providing dysphagia treatment

Multidisciplinary approach	A team of professionals from different disciplines who independently treat patients from their own perspective and formally interact with little or no awareness of the work of professionals from other disciplines.
Interdisciplinary approach	A team of professionals from diverse fields who work in a coordinated manner toward a common goal for the patient. Information is exchanged and communicated, and a consensus regarding the treatment plan is established among team members, typically during team meetings.
Transdisciplinary approach	A team composed of professionals from various fields cooperating across disciplines and has flexibility for the diversity of team composition. Disciplinary boundaries are blurred; team members share roles to achieve broader and deeper analysis, leading to a more efficiently integrated team approach.

Physiatrists play an important role in the treatment-oriented evaluation and management of dysphagia using videoendoscopy (VE) and VF to perform swallowing examinations.

In Japan, dentists also play a major role in the field of dysphagia rehabilitation by using VE and VF to evaluate swallowing function and diagnose swallowing disorders. Moreover, dentists and dental hygienists work together in the care and treatment of oral health problems to improve eating function and reduce the risk of aspiration pneumonia.

Otolaryngologists closely cooperate as necessary in both research and surgical treatment of severe dysphagia.

SLHTs mainly perform dysphagia rehabilitation in the form of intensive exercise.

Certified dysphagia nurses play a primary role in patient screening, integration and collaboration with professionals in other disciplines, and eating function therapy. In addition, assessment of patients' activities of daily living (ADL) is necessary to determine their task performance ability and need for assistance by a caregiver.

The team members meet weekly in a conference to discuss their interpretations of patients' findings and possible directions for further interventions. Treatment plans are made, and treatment outcomes are followed in these conferences. In addition to clinical care, the team contributes to scientific discussions on swallowing disorders to enhance and encourage the dissemination of knowledge derived from research of dysphagia.

References

1. Puisieux F, D'andrea C, Baconnier P, Bui-Dinh D, Castaings-Pelet S, Crestani B, et al. Swallowing disorders, pneumonia and respiratory tract infectious disease in the elderly. Rev Mal Respir. 2009;26:587–605.
2. Logemann JA, Curro FA, Pauloski B, Gensler G. Aging effects on oropharyngeal swallow and the role of dental care in oropharyngeal dysphagia. Oral Dis. 2013;19(8):733–7. doi:10.1111/odi.12104.

3. Kuroda Y. Relationship between swallowing function, and functional and nutritional status in hospitalized elderly individuals. Int J Speech Lang Pathol Audiol. 2014;2:20–6.
4. Clavé P, Shaker R. Dysphagia: current reality and scope of the problem. Nat Rev Gastroenterol Hepatol. 2015;12(5):259–70. doi:10.1038/nrgastro.2015.49.
5. Wirth R, Dziewas R, Beck AM, Clavé P, Hamdy S, Heppner HJ, et al. Oropharyngeal dysphagia in older persons - from pathophysiology to adequate intervention: a review and summary of an international expert meeting. Clin Interv Aging. 2016;11:189–208. doi:10.2147/CIA.S97481.
6. Sura L, Madhavan A, Carnaby G, Crary MA. Dysphagia in the elderly: management and nutritional considerations. Clin Interv Aging. 2012;7:287–98. doi:10.2147/CIA.S23404.
7. Martino R, Foley N, Bhogal S, Diamant N, Speechley M, Teasell R. Dysphagia after stroke: incidence, diagnosis, and pulmonary complications. Stroke. 2005;36(12):2756–63.
8. Martino R, Martin RE, Black S. Dysphagia after stroke and its management. CMAJ. 2012;184(10):1127–8. doi:10.1503/cmaj.101659.
9. Carrión S, Cabré M, Monteis R, Roca M, Palomera E, Serra-Prat M, et al. Oropharyngeal dysphagia is a prevalent risk factor for malnutrition in a cohort of older patients admitted with an acute disease to a general hospital. Clin Nutr. 2015;34(3):436–42. doi:10.1016/j.clnu.2014.04.014.
10. Maeshima S, Osawa A, Miyazaki Y, Seki Y, Miura C, Tazawa Y, et al. Influence of dysphagia on short-term outcome in patients with acute stroke. Am J Phys Med Rehabil. 2011;90(4):316–20. doi:10.1097/PHM.0b013e31820b13b2.
11. Guyomard V, Fulcher RA, Redmayne O, Metcalf AK, Potter JF, Myint PK. Effect of dysphasia and dysphagia on inpatient mortality and hospital length of stay: a database study. J Am Geriatr Soc. 2009;57(11):2101–6. doi:10.1111/j.1532-5415.2009.02526.x.
12. Altman KW, Yu GP, Schaefer SD. Consequence of dysphagia in the hospitalized patient: impact on prognosis and hospital resources. Arch Otolaryngol Head Neck Surg. 2010;136(8):784–9. doi:10.1001/archoto.2010.129.
13. Martens L, Cameron T, Simonsen M. Effects of a multidisciplinary management program on neurologically impaired patients with dysphagia. Dysphagia. 1990;5(3):147–51.
14. Farneti D, Consolmagno P. The swallowing centre: rationale for a multidisciplinary management. Acta Otorhinolaryngol Ital. 2007;27(4):200–7.
15. Aoki S, Hosomi N, Hirayama J, Nakamori M, Yoshikawa M, Nezu T, et al. The multidisciplinary swallowing team approach decreases pneumonia onset in acute stroke patients. PLoS One. 2016;11(5):e0154608. doi:10.1371/journal.pone.0154608.
16. Saitoh E, Matsuo K, Inamoto Y, Ishikawa M, Tsubahara A. Twenty years of trans-disciplinary approach development for dysphagia rehabilitation in Japan. Dysphagia. 2015;30(1):102–3. doi:10.1007/s00455-014-9591-0.
17. Toda F, Kagaya H, Baba M, Shibata S, Ozeki Y, Kanamori D, et al. Effect of swallowing rounds on the outcome of dysphagic patients. Jpn J Compr Rehabil Sci. 2015;6:50–5.

Chapter 5
Clinical Evaluation of Dysphagia

Kannit Pongpipatpaiboon, Yoko Inamoto, Yoichiro Aoyagi, Seiko Shibata, Hitoshi Kagaya, and Koichiro Matsuo

Abstract Clinical evaluation, both instrumental and noninstrumental, plays an important role in the swallowing assessment of the patients with dysphagia. The gathered information from thorough evaluation contributes the presence of dysphagia, dysphagia severity level, rehabilitation planning, and both the problem and the potential solution. The dysphagia screening, clinical and instrumental assessment, and new perspectives in advanced swallowing assessment will be described in this chapter.

Dysphagia is a complication commonly associated with cerebrovascular accidents and occurs within 3 days of the cerebrovascular accident in approximately 42–67% of patients [1]. Cerebral and brain stem strokes are the main cause of swallowing disorders. Dysphagia tends to have a greater likelihood of recovery after hemispheric stroke because of the plasticity and compensatory reorganization in the contralateral motor cortex. Conversely, dysphagia in patients with brain stem stroke is more likely to remain prominent. Dysphagia contributes to a greater risk of aspiration and pneumonia ranging in severity from the need for outpatient treatment to death. Stroke patients with dysphagia, regardless of its severity or the presence of aspiration, are approximately three times more likely to develop pneumonia than are patients without dysphagia [2].

K. Pongpipatpaiboon • Y. Aoyagi • S. Shibata • H. Kagaya
Department of Rehabilitation Medicine I, School of Medicine, Fujita Health University, Toyoake, Aichi, Japan
e-mail: ning665@gmail.com; yyy@rc5.so-net.ne.jp; sshibata@fujita-hu.ac.jp; hkagaya2@fujita-hu.ac.jp

Y. Inamoto (✉)
Faculty of Rehabilitation, School of Health Sciences, Fujita Health University, 1-98 Dengakugakubo, Kutsukake, Toyoake, Aichi 470-1192, Japan
e-mail: inamoto@fujita-hu.ac.jp

K. Matsuo
Department of Dentistry, School of Medicine, Fujita Health University, Toyoake, Aichi, Japan
e-mail: kmatsuo@fujita-hu.ac.jp

E. Saitoh et al. (eds.), *Dysphagia Evaluation and Treatment*,
https://doi.org/10.1007/978-981-10-5032-9_5

Emerging evidences have shown that early identification of dysphagia and the risk of aspiration can help to reduce adverse health consequences such as pulmonary complications, dehydration, and malnutrition; shorten the hospital stay; and reduce overall healthcare costs [3–6]. Positive changes in health outcomes indicate that early and reliable screening of patients at risk of swallowing disorders is a vital first step in effective and appropriate dysphagia management. Clinical screening methods with which to identify patients who require referral for further swallowing functional evaluation, including videofluorography (VF), are essential.

The basic parameters in a swallowing evaluation are the patient's performance status (including consciousness level and respiratory status), intellectual function, oropharyngeal structure and function, level of ADL, caregiver use, and available resources.

Basic evaluation should be in the following order before planning further management, including dysphagia screening, instrumental swallowing assessment, and clinical swallowing assessment.

The presence or absence of dysphagia is first determined using screening tests. Further evaluation using techniques such as VF, videoendoscopy (VE), or others is then performed if the screening test failed and more details of diagnosis are needed to achieve a diagnosis. Upon completion of a comprehensive evaluation, the level of the patient's swallowing dysfunction with quantification of aspiration is determined with the Dysphagia Severity Scale (DSS) [7] to summarize the functional problem (Table 5.1). Additionally, the patient's eating condition is determined using the Eating Status Scale (ESS) (Table 5.2). The patient's medical stability is determined to be unstable or stable, where stable means no signs of dehydration, malnutrition, or pneumonia found by observations performed every 2 weeks.

Both the DSS and ESS are correlated with each other and important for treatment planning, including making recommendations regarding the diet level, independence

Table 5.1 Function severity score of dysphagia using the Dysphagia Severity Scale, a seven-point ordinal scale

Severity score	Definition	Characteristics
7	Within normal limits	No condition of dysphagia
6	Minimum problem	Some symptoms of dysphagia but no need of rehabilitation or exercise
5	Oral problem	Significant symptoms of oral preparatory or oral stage without aspiration
4	Occasional aspiration	Possible aspiration or aspiration is suspected due to much pharyngeal residue
3	Water aspiration	Aspiration of thin liquid. Changes in food consistency will be effective
2	Food aspiration	Food aspiration with no effect of compensatory techniques or food consistency changes
1	Saliva aspiration	Unstable medical condition because of severe saliva aspiration

Table 5.2 Eating Status Scale, a five-point ordinal

Score	Characteristics
5	Oral feeding
4	Modified oral feeding
3	Oral > tube
2	Oral < tube
1	Tube feeding only

level, interventions, management plan, and the monitoring of swallowing improvement after exercise therapy.

These scales are helpful in comparing the level of swallowing dysfunction within and across patients and reevaluating swallowing impairment with respect to treatment effectiveness. Use of the DSS in conjunction with the ESS is essential. Although swallowing function (assessed with the DSS) is not altered during reexamination, the eating status (assessed with the ESS) can demonstrate improvement if safe swallowing and a decrease in the risk of aspiration are achieved by appropriate food adjustment.

5.1 Dysphagia Screening

Evaluation of swallowing in patients who present to the hospital with swallowing dysfunction begins with screening. The screening of swallowing function is a rapid procedure with the purpose of identifying patients at risk for oropharyngeal dysphagia. Screening should be applied as soon as the patient's medical condition allows, to guide further assessment and determine whether the patient can safely take food by mouth. Clinicians should understand the importance of this screening and remember that it cannot be used to diagnose dysphagia.

Depending on the setting, screening can be conducted by a physician, nurse, or SLHT. Additionally, various screening tests are used in different work settings. No single dysphagia screening tool can be regarded as the most effective and ready for complete clinical implementation [2, 8].

Patients who undergo a failed initial screening require referral for both clinical (noninstrumental) and instrumental swallow assessments. These evaluations allow clinicians to obtain a more comprehensive, in-depth understanding of the swallow physiology; determine the presence, location, and severity of the impairment; and plan further management.

Screening tools need to involve easy-to-perform protocols, few time-consuming procedures, and noninvasive methods with which to determine the risk of dysphagia and/or aspiration. Above all, the screening tool must have proven reliability and validity [9, 10] for use in the clinical setting. Additionally, because the aim of screening tools is to identify patients at greater risk of dysphagia, these tools must also have high sensitivity and a low rate of false-negative results.

Several dysphagia screening tools are used in Japan. The main screening tests performed on a routine basis at FHUR are described below.

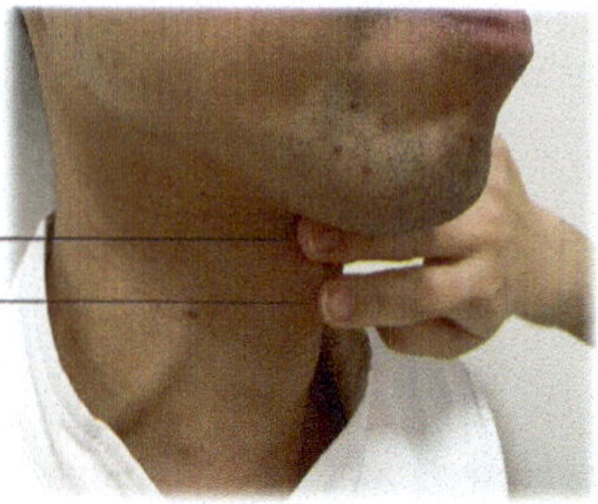

Fig. 5.1 The examiner places the index and middle fingers on the hyoid bone and thyroid cartilage, respectively, during the repetitive saliva swallowing test

5.1.1 *Repetitive Saliva Swallowing Test*

The repetitive saliva swallowing test (RSST) was developed to safely and simply screen patients with functional dysphagia. It detects the patient's ability to voluntarily swallow repeatedly and correlates the results with the risk of aspiration. The patient stays in a resting posture and is asked to repeatedly swallow saliva (dry swallow) as many times as possible within 30 s. The examiner counts the number of swallows by palpation or inspection of laryngeal elevation movement during the swallowing reflex (Fig. 5.1). A patient with two or fewer dry swallows within 30 s is likely to have dysphagia associated with aspiration and should be further investigated.

The sensitivity and specificity of the RSST to detect aspiration diagnosed using VF as reference test are 0.98 and 0.66, respectively [11, 12]. However, the RSST has limited clinical applicability in patients with cognitive or linguistic dysfunction because these patients may lack the ability to follow instructions.

5.1.2 *Modified Water Swallowing Test*

The modified water swallowing test (MWST) is used to detect aspiration when swallowing water and monitoring the response. A 3-mL volume of cold water is placed on the floor of the mouth with a syringe, and the patient is instructed to swallow the water followed by two saliva swallows (Fig. 5.2). If the patient is unable to swallow or experiences dyspnea, coughing, or wet-hoarse dysphonia after swallowing, a score of 1–3 is recorded and the test is terminated. If the patient is able to swallow the water safely, a score of 4 or 5 is recorded depending on the patient's ability to perform the two dry swallows afterward.

Breathing, coughing, and voice quality are scored using a five-point scale (Table 5.3).

The entire procedure is repeated twice more. The final score is determined as the lowest score of any trial. This test is an easy, simple, and safe method with which to evaluate swallowing function.

The sensitivity and specificity of the MWST to detect aspiration using VF for concurrent validity are 0.70 and 0.88, respectively, when the cutoff score is 3 [13, 14].

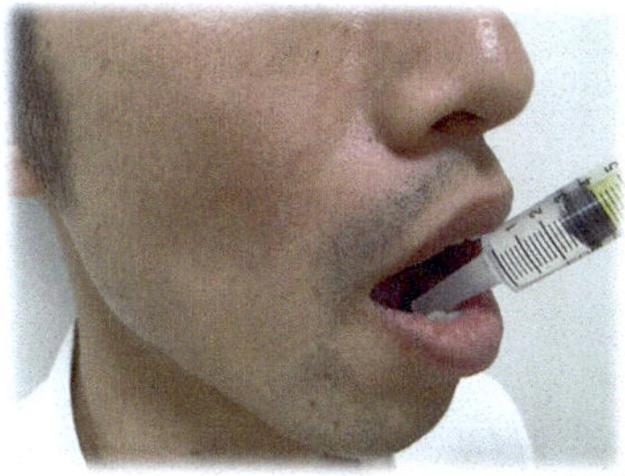

Fig. 5.2 The examiner places 3 mL of water into the mouth (under the tongue) with a syringe during the modified water swallowing test

Table 5.3 Scoring system for modified water swallowing test

Score	Characters
1	No swallow, cough, and/or frequent breathing
2	Swallowed successfully without coughing but with changes in breathing (e.g., frequent breathing)
3	Swallowed successfully with normal breathing but with cough and/or wet-hoarse voice
4	Swallowed successfully with normal breathing, no cough, and no wet-hoarse voice
5	Score 4, plus two or more additional dry swallows in 30 s

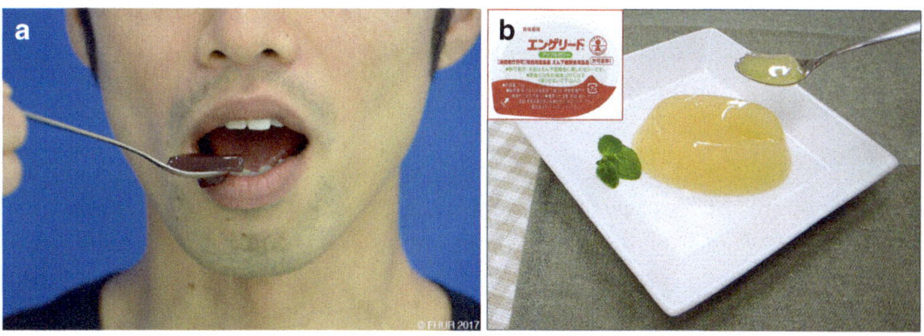

Fig. 5.3 (**a**) The examiner places a 4-g bolus of jelly into the mouth with a spoon during the food test. (**b**) Pudding or jelly may be used for the food test ((**b**) Reproduced from Otsuka Pharmaceutical Factory, Inc. with permission)

5.1.3 Food Test

The food test is a modification developed to screen for solid food dysphagia. The procedure and scoring are nearly identical to those of the MWST. A 4-g bolus of pudding or jelly is placed on the dorsum of the tongue with a spoon, and the patient is then instructed to swallow. In addition to scoring the components of MWST, oral residue after swallowing must be inspected (Fig. 5.3; Table 5.4).

Table 5.4 Scoring system for food test

Score	Characters
1	No swallow, cough, and/or frequent breathing
2	Swallowed successfully without coughing but with changes in breathing (e.g., frequent breathing)
3	Swallowed successfully with normal breathing but with cough and/or wet-hoarse voice and/or moderate residue in oral cavity
4	Swallowed successfully with normal breathing, no cough, no wet-hoarse voice, and almost no residue in oral cavity
5	Score 4, plus two or more additional dry swallows in 30 s

Table 5.5 Scoring system for 30-mL water swallowing test

Score	Characters
1	Drink all the water in one gulp without choking
2	Drink all the water in two or more gulps without choking
3	Drink all the water in one gulp but with some choking
4	Drink all the water in two or more gulps but with some choking
5	Chokes and has difficulty drinking all the water

The sensitivity and specificity of the food test to detect aspiration as diagnosed by VF are 0.72 and 0.62, respectively, when the cutoff score is 4 [14].

5.1.4 30-mL Water Swallowing Test

The 30-mL water swallowing test (WST) was originally described by Kubota [15, 16] using 30 mL of water at room temperature to detect aspiration. The patient is asked to drink water from the cup in the sitting position as usual. The drinking profile is based on a five-point scale, and the occurrence of drinking episodes (described below) and duration of drinking are monitored and assessed (Table 5.5).

5.1.4.1 Drinking Episodes

Examples of drinking episodes include sipping, holding water in the mouth while drinking, escape of water from the mouth, a tendency to try to force himself/herself to continue drinking despite choking, and drinking water in a cautious manner.

5.1.4.2 Diagnosis

Normal: Completed Profile 1 within 5 s
Suspected aspiration: Completed Profile 1 in more than 5 s or completed Profile 2
Abnormal: Completed any of Profiles 3 through 5

Nevertheless, because of the high risk of aspiration in patients with stroke and older individuals swallowing large amounts of water, the above-described 3-mL MWST was developed for use on the first attempt; this is followed by the 30-mL WST (Fig. 5.4).

Notably, the laryngeal movement, timing/completeness/number of swallows, pre–post-voice quality, coughing/throat clearing, absent or delayed swallowing, and oral residue should be observed and recorded during all trial swallows.

At the FHUR, a certified nurse of dysphagia nursing is the main person who administers the swallowing screening test to patients who are at risk of dysphagia or are suspected to have dysphagia. Figure 5.5 shows a diagram of dysphagia screening executed by a certified nurse of dysphagia nursing at the FHUR.

Safety is an important consideration. A pulse oximeter for monitoring the arterial oxygen saturation, tools for clinical observation, and a suction unit should be ready in case they are needed during the swallow test. Furthermore, these screening tests

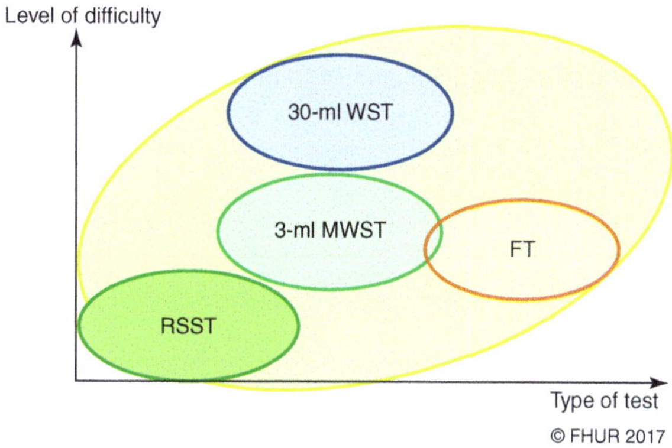

Fig. 5.4 Degree of test difficulty. *The accuracy of the screening result can be increased by the combination of different screening tests

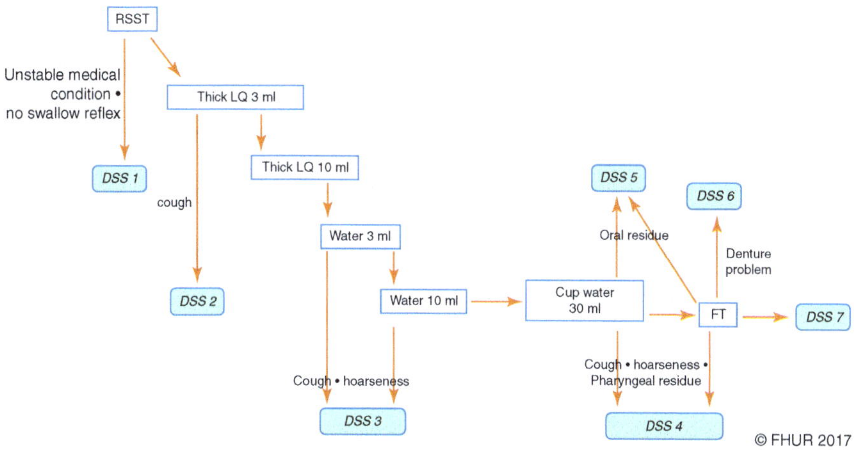

Fig. 5.5 Guideline of dysphagia screening tests in FHUR. The Dysphagia Severity Scale is used to determine the severity of swallowing dysfunction during the swallowing screening

may not detect silent (subclinical) aspiration and cannot always provide information that is useful for treatment.

Other than the screening tests used at FHUR, a large amount of emerging evidence shows that dysphagia screening tools are sensitive, specific, and easily administered without extensive training (Appendix). Moreover, dysphagia screening can alternatively be performed with the use of questionnaires, which are being increasingly used to collect data that quantify the symptomatic severity of dysphagia as experienced by the patient. These questionnaires also have evidence supporting their clinical use (e.g., the ten-item Eating Assessment Tool, Seirei Questionnaire of Swallowing, Swallow Disturbance Questionnaire).

Another step after screening is a more comprehensive assessment. Patients with suspected dysphagia or who are at high risk of dysphagia require further assessment after the screening test has failed.

Swallowing assessment after screening encompasses a clinical swallow assessment and instrumental measures. The combination of clinical and instrumental measures contributes to a more comprehensive understanding of the patient's swallowing problem, allowing the clinician to gather useful information for a proper diagnosis and individualized treatment planning. The diagram below illustrates a holistic approach for patients with suspected or confirmed dysphagia (Fig. 5.6).

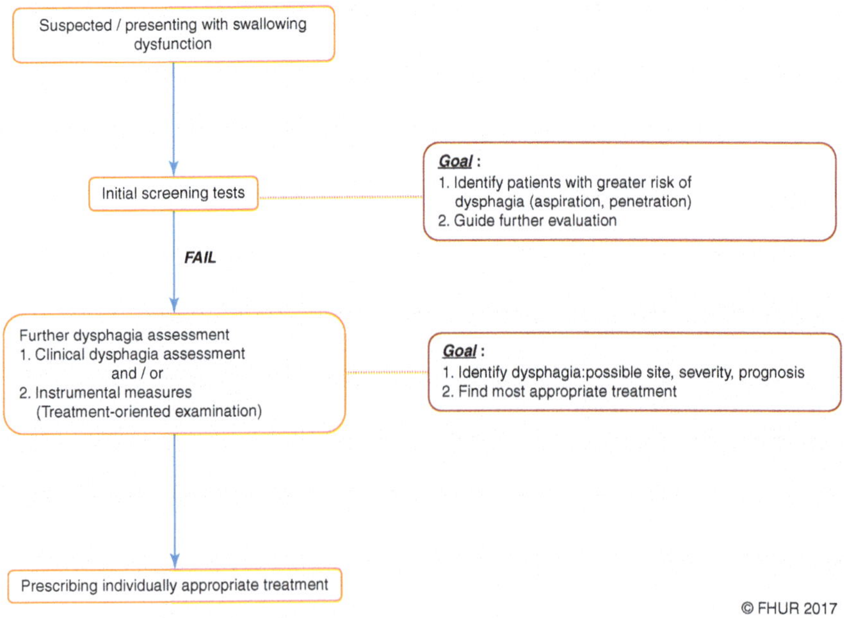

Fig. 5.6 Evaluation of patients with suspected dysphagia

5.2 Clinical Swallowing Assessment

A positive (failed) screening result is followed by a clinical swallowing examination. This pathway is very useful in centers with sufficient amounts of clinicians and equipment, like the FHUR. Alternatively, a clinical swallowing examination can be performed before further evaluation or instrumental examination in small centers with a shortage of human resources and/or equipment.

The clinical swallowing assessment serves to validate and identify the severity of dysphagia and guide further management. The main objectives of the evaluation are problem recognition, identification of the pathophysiology involved, and acquisition of data to determine the etiology of the condition.

This information is gathered to gain a more holistic view of the patient, make decisions on his or her swallowing ability, and make predictions regarding the presence or absence of dysphagia and aspiration. Thorough history-taking and physical examination, including medication use, is essential to determine the etiology of dysphagia. Swallowing is a complex process, and dysphagia may result from abnormalities in any of the many steps necessary for deglutition. These various causes can be classified by patient age range or pathophysiology. The pathophysiologic disorders causing dysphagia can be categorized as shown in Table 5.6.

The pie chart in Fig. 5.7 shows the etiologies of VF-diagnosed dysphagia among 275 patients at FHUR in 2016. The average age of the patients was 66 ± 19 years (range, 10.8 months to 97 years). Poststroke dysphagia was the most common etiologies of dysphagia.

Table 5.6 Major categories of various disorders causing dysphagia

Neuromuscular disorders	• Central nervous system diseases (such as stroke, Parkinson disease), multiple cranial nerve palsy, bulbar palsy (e.g., multiple sclerosis, motor neuron disease) • Myasthenia gravis, muscular dystrophy, etc.
Mechanical and obstructive disorders	• Head and neck malignancy and their consequences of surgery and/or radiotherapeutic interventions • Acute inflammation or infections (e.g., retropharyngeal abscesses) • Zenker diverticulum • Cervical osteophytes • Fibrosis/cricopharyngeal bar • Tracheostomy, etc.
Esophageal disorders	• Structural disorders (tumors, eosinophilic esophagitis, infections, radiation injury, esophageal rings and webs, etc.) • Dysmotility (achalasia, esophageal spasm, scleroderma, connective tissue disease (e.g., myositis)) • Gastroesophageal reflux disease
Others	• Drug-induced, psychogenic, age-related changes, major categories of head and neck disorders causing dysphagia

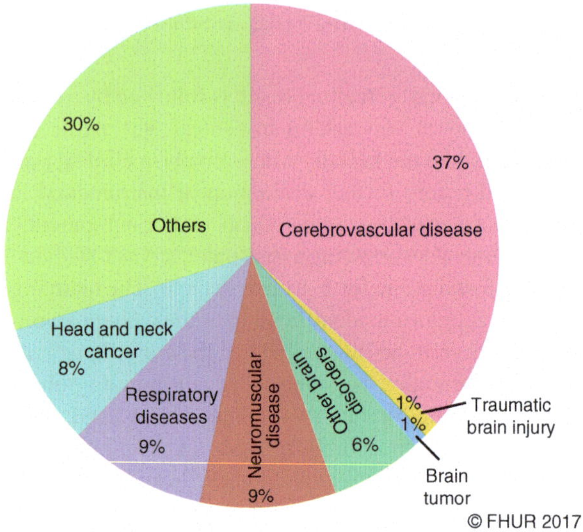

Fig. 5.7 Etiologies of swallowing disorders diagnosed by VF at FHUR in 2016

The most efficient and precise technique with which to identify dysphagia requires a thorough comprehensive evaluation of the patient's medical history and a complete physical examination.

5.2.1 Medical History

A comprehensive history must include the information shown in Table 5.7.

This information is ideally obtained directly from the patient. However, when the patient is unable to provide this information because of a limited cognitive status or language restriction, the history of the swallowing problem is acquired and validated by the patient's family or caregiver, the medical team, and/or the medical record. Knowledge of the potential etiology of the dysphagia is critical. A curable or ameliorating etiology, such as infection or stroke, respectively, can suggest the potential to improve the patient's swallowing ability. Conversely, a progressive disease such as a neurodegenerative disease or amyotrophic lateral sclerosis suggests a poor swallowing prognosis over time. This information affects the ability to establish a feasible and appropriate treatment plan.

5.2.2 Physical Examination

It is important to assess the patient's physical findings in terms of both structure and function. This assessment consists of various general assessments (described below) and evaluation of the cranial nerves, particularly cranial nerves V, VII, IX, X, and XII because these are strongly associated with the motor and sensory functions of swallowing.

Table 5.7 Medical history required for diagnosis

Patient presenting symptoms	• Difficulty initiating a swallow, repetitive swallowing • Take extra effort to swallow liquids/solids/pills • Changes of tastes • Nasal speech, nasal regurgitation • Drooling • Coughing and/or choking (before, during, or after swallowing) • Globus pharyngeus (feeling of food stuck in the throat) • Painful swallow • Dysarthria • Wet hoarseness (gurgling voice) • Changes voice/speech after swallow • Changes in breathing when eating or drinking • Increasing secretion • Halitosis • Weight loss, etc.
Past history and current medical status	• Diagnosis of neurological diseases (e.g., stroke, Parkinson disease, myasthenia gravis, cranial nerve-involved diseases) • Other underlying diseases accompanying dysphagia or related to possible coexisting swallowing disorders (e.g., head and neck cancer, chronic obstructive pulmonary disease, congestive heart failure, gastrointestinal diseases) • Dental disorder and previous treatment
Current medication	• Anticholinergics, antipsychotics, tricyclic antidepressants, antiepileptic drugs, skeletal muscle relaxants, sedative drugs, etc.
Specific swallowing history	• Onset, duration, and course of problem: gradually worse in case of neurological disorders in particular • Weight loss, loss of appetite • History of recent and recurrent pneumonia • Eating condition: oral/dental status, feeding dependency, difficult food/liquid items, length of meal time taken, precipitating or alleviating factors, episodes and frequency of choking/coughing, drooling/difficulty of saliva swallowing, energy level • Previous swallowing assessment (intervention and treatment provided)
Sociocultural status	• Cultural background, personal and environmental support

5.2.2.1 General Assessments

The four primary areas of examination in the general assessments are:

1. Mental status
   - Alertness/wakefulness, cooperation, orientation, and communication
2. Nutritional status
   - Type of feeding, signs of dehydration, signs of malnutrition, and body mass index

3. Respiratory status

   - Respiratory rate, arterial oxygen saturation, breathing patterns, ability to hold breathing, and difficulty of breathing
   - Chest auscultation
   - Weakness of voluntary cough
   - Presence of tracheostomy and type of tracheostomy tube
   - Saliva aspiration and the presence of secretion
   - Suction equipment

4. Oral healthcare and dentition

   - Oral hygiene, oral mucosa (moist/dry), food residue, dentures, tooth decay, mucositis/gingivitis, etc.

In addition, postural control (ability to maintain the sitting position), mobility function, ambulatory level, and requirement of assistance should be assessed.

5.2.2.2 Assessment of Oromotor Control and Vocal Function

- Jaw movement, labial function, and cheek and facial movement
- Lingual function (at rest and during movement)
- Soft palate and pharynx: weakness, asymmetry, and sensation of the posterior pharyngeal wall
- Laryngeal function

  - Vocal quality (normal, hoarseness, wet/gurgling voice)
  - Volitional cough (strong, weak, absent)
  - Throat clearing (strong, weak, absent)
  - Phonation time (seconds)

- Others: dysarthria, oral apraxia, laryngeal elevation, and reflexes (gag reflex, bite reflex)

The evaluation guidelines proposed by the JSDR in 2011 suggest the need to clinically evaluate the patient with respect to at least eight items:

1. Cognition
2. Observation of eating
3. Range of motion of the head and neck
4. Dental prosthesis and oral hygiene
5. Oral motor and sensory examination
6. Phonation and articulation
7. Pulmonary function
8. Nutrition and hydration

Clinical diagnosis of dysphagia in Japan is performed by physiatrists, SLHTs, and nurses. Nevertheless, it is important to note that the clinical swallowing examination has several limitations. It cannot be used to identify the underlying swallowing impairment, confirm airway invasion, determine the effects of compensatory strategies, or recommend appropriate rehabilitation approaches. Instead, an instrumental swallowing evaluation (VF and/or VE) is warranted for these purposes and should be implemented.

5.3 Instrumental Swallowing Assessment

The instrumental swallowing assessment helps the clinician to identify the biomechanical aspects of the patient's swallowing dysfunction, determine the risk of aspiration, assess the patient's compensatory strategies, and make swallowing rehabilitation training recommendations through the appropriate use and interpretation of a diagnostic swallow procedure. Instrumental swallowing assessment involves any or all of the following procedures to examine a particular aspect of swallowing. Such assessment not only provides valuable information with which to achieve a clinical diagnosis but also facilitates establishment of the most appropriate swallowing rehabilitation training program.

- Assessment of structural and functional swallow
- Assessment of adequacy of airway protection
- Assessment of coordination of respiration and swallowing
- Screening of esophageal motility and gastroesophageal regurgitation
- Assessment of the effects of changes in bolus delivery, changes in bolus characteristics (consistency and volume), and compensatory swallowing strategies using therapeutic postures or maneuvers

Aspiration is concerning because it can lead to aspiration pneumonia or pulmonary disease, which can be fatal in many cases. Therefore, accurate assessment of aspiration and identification of pathophysiology under aspiration is essential.

An instrumental swallowing assessment is indicated to achieve the correct diagnosis and plan appropriate management that ensures safe and effective swallowing in patients who have dysphagia or are at high risk of developing dysphagia when:

- Signs and symptoms are not consistent with the clinical examination findings.
- Further detailed information is needed to determine the most likely diagnosis or underlying swallowing impairment.
- The safety and efficiency of the swallow are being assessed.
- Compensatory strategies are being assessed, and the most appropriate rehabilitation protocol is being individually recommended, including behavioral and dietary management.
- The swallow function changes after treatment, or the patient has a chronic degenerative disease that is known to gradually progress.

The two main swallowing diagnostic tools are VF and VE. Both procedures are considered to be the gold standard techniques for swallowing evaluation because they are outstanding treatment-oriented tools and have undergone evidence-based validation. Which procedure is needed for a swallow evaluation is determined by individual patient characteristics and the purpose of the evaluation.

5.3.1 Swallowing Examination by Videofluorography (VF)

Swallowing examination using VF is a treatment-oriented evaluation that provides real-time visualization of the bolus trajectory in the oral cavity, oropharynx, hypopharynx, and esophagus using various consistencies and volumes of barium-coated trial materials.

VF has been proposed as the gold standard assessment method with which to establish a standard for image evaluation and is considered a mandatory tool for swallowing evaluation. It allows for a kinematic evaluation during the study and a more detailed kinematic analysis using the recorded image after the study, contributing to the establishment of a treatment plan.

VF provides two essential feedback parameters for treatment: knowledge of results and knowledge of performance. Knowledge of results is the feedback regarding whether aspiration and/or residue is present. Knowledge of performance is the feedback regarding how to eliminate this aspiration/residue. Thus, for knowledge of results, identifying the least difficulty task that can prevent aspiration and/or residue is essential, and for knowledge of performance, detecting the tip to eliminate aspiration and/or residue is essential. Determining appropriate food modification, postural techniques, and swallowing maneuvers as the least difficulty task and tip are the basis of evaluation. VF also allows the clinician to assess the availability, adequacy, and effect of the intervention in terms of reaching the treatment goal.

Four evaluation points are important when performing VF:

- Handling bolus in mouth (chewing, bolus formation, bolus propelling)
- Position of the bolus head
- Evidence of aspiration/penetration (before, during, or after swallow)
- Volume and location of the oral and/or pharyngeal residue

The results of these evaluations will help to determine the most effective strategies (e.g., bolus modification or postural techniques during VF) that ensure efficient and safe swallowing. Other details should also be observed depending on the individual patient's problems.

Laryngeal penetration and the risk of aspiration associated with the bolus type are observed while performing VF. The order of the tests is not fixed; the clinician adapts the examination to the individual patient. The clinician can select the bolus materials depending on the patient's swallowing impairment and complaints about foods that are difficult to swallow. According to the differences between eating and drinking, clinicians should evaluate both of these behaviors in terms of the chew–swallow complex. One study demonstrated that the act of chewing was a prime determining factor of the chew–swallow complex during stage II transport of the process model [17].

As seen in Fig. 5.8, the two-phase food (mixed food) is associated with the highest risk of aspiration because the bolus head is significantly lower in the food pathway at swallowing onset than either liquid or corned beef hash. The leading edge of the two-phase food reaches the vallecula or a lower area of the hypopharynx before swallowing onset. This means that the patient's chewing manner influences the depth of the leading edge of the bolus at the onset of pharyngeal swallow. This occurs even when drinking liquid by performing chewing. Clinicians should therefore assess the chew–swallow complex in addition to performing conventional VF, and a two-phase food should be used to evaluate the risk of aspiration (Table 5.8).

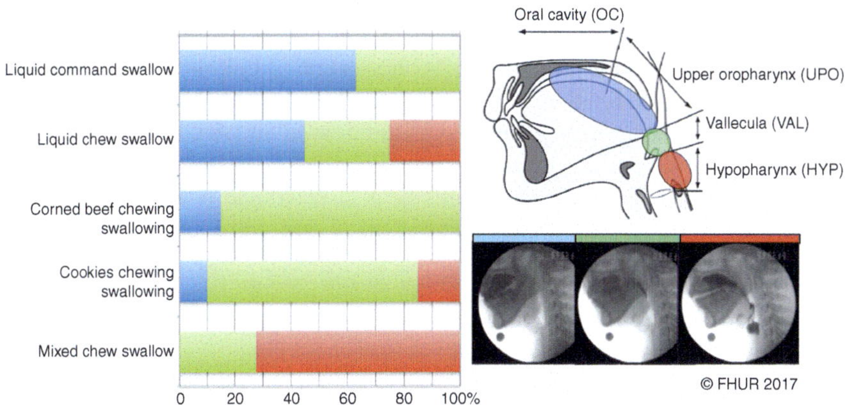

Fig. 5.8 The bolus position at the time of the swallowing onset based on the bolus characteristics. A mixed chew–swallow refers to a two-phase food comprising liquid barium and corned beef hash. *This was the result of ten healthy subjects (six male, four female; age, 29 ± 4 years) using 10 mL of liquid barium, 8 g of corned beef hash, 8 g of cookie, and a bolus of mixed consistency (4 g of corned beef hash and 5 mL of liquid barium)

Table 5.8 Paired comparisons to determine risk of aspiration among various types of foods and drinks [18]

	PD	CB	LQ4	LQ10	CUP	MX
PD		○	○	○	○	○
CB	●		○	○	○	○
LQ4	●	●		○	○	○
LQ10	●	●	●		○	○
CUP	●	●	●	●		○
MX	●	●	●	●	●	

● More likely to cause aspiration
○ Less likely to cause aspiration

PD pudding-thick texture, *CB* corned beef hash, *LQ4* 4 mL of thin liquid, *LQ10* 10 mL of thin liquid, *CUP* one swallow from a cup, *MX* two-phase mixture of 4 g of corned beef hash and 5 mL of thin liquid

Patients with dysphagia should be assessed with caution when eating multi-textured food to clarify the most appropriate bolus types for each patient. Prepared bolus materials should be initially tested from the safest and easiest to the most difficult materials, and the patient should begin the examination using a small amount of liquid barium or a small bolus of food to enable safe assessment of the patient's basic swallow physiology and clarification of further management. If the bolus can still be safely swallowed after modification of its consistency and volume, the study proceeds by administration of the next bolus with a higher risk of aspiration (more difficult task). This step-by-step administration is continued until the clinician detects the task that results in aspiration. Various foods and liquids that differ in volume, consistency, and texture are used. Liquid barium is administered by syringe for 4- and 10-mL boluses placed under the tongue and by cup or straw for 30-g boluses to observe sequential drinking. **The patient is asked to hold the bolus in his or her mouth until instructed to swallow.

In addition to modification of the boluses administered during VF, postural techniques (e.g., head rotation, trunk rotation, reclining posture, head/neck flexion) and swallowing maneuvers (e.g., super-supraglottic swallow, Mendelsohn maneuver, Effortful swallow) can be utilized to enhance safety and facilitate selection of appropriate treatment. These procedures help to determine how to improve the oropharyngeal swallow and return the patient to full oral intake as quickly as possible (Table 5.9).

Table 5.9 Summary of common bolus materials, postural techniques, and therapeutic maneuvers used during videofluorography

Various foods and liquids • Volume 2 mL and then go further with 4 mL, 10 mL, and cup drinking (30 g) • Bolus – Thin liquid, nectar-thickened liquid, and honey-thickened liquid – Semisolid, solid food, and two-phase food (chew–swallow)
Posture strategies • Head and/or neck flexion (chin tuck) • Head rotation • Reclining • Trunk rotation
Swallowing maneuvers • Effortful swallow • Mendelsohn maneuver • Supraglottic swallow • Super-supraglottic swallow • Etc.

Table 5.10 Key features observed in the lateral and anteroposterior fluoroscopic views

Lateral view	AP view
Boundaries of lateral fluoroscopic view • Nasopharynx superiorly • Cervical esophagus inferiorly (below UES) • Lip anteriorly • Cervical spine posteriorly	*Boundaries of AP fluoroscopic view* • Nasopharynx superiorly • Cervical esophagus inferiorly (below UES) • Lateral pharyngeal walls
Point of view: structural movement • Lip closure • Tongue motion – Base of tongue retraction – Squeeze back • Soft palate elevation • Epiglottis inversion • Pharyngeal contraction • UES opening	*Point of view: structural movement* • Tongue motion – Tongue rotation – Mastication – Food transport • Pharyngeal contraction • Symmetry of bolus trajectory • UES opening • Esophageal motion
Bolus flow trajectory and functional abnormalities • Leakage from lip (drooling) • Poor bolus formation and transfer • Premature spillage • Penetration/aspiration (before, during, after swallowing) • Impaired pharyngo-laryngeal elevation • Residue (oral, pharynx, vallecular, pyriform sinuses) – Amount – Location – Patient response • Nasal/pharyngeal regurgitation	*Bolus flow trajectory and functional abnormalities* • Tongue motion weakness • Poor bolus formation and transfer • Impaired pharyngo-laryngeal elevation • Impaired pharyngeal contraction • Laterality of bolus flow (asymmetrical property) • Residue located side • Incompetent esophageal peristalsis • Slow esophageal transit through the esophagus • Esophago-pharyngeal regurgitation and gastroesophageal regurgitation

The most important image of the swallowing study is the lateral view, which enables observation of the movement of the tongue base, soft palate elevation, hyolaryngeal elevation, laryngeal closure, contraction of the pharyngeal constrictor, and opening of the upper esophageal sphincter (UES). However, the anteroposterior view must also be assessed because it provides important clinical information regarding the pharyngeal constriction, the laterality of bolus flow (symmetrical characteristic), the side on which the pharyngeal residue is located, and anatomical abnormalities such as pharyngeal diverticula. This view also allows for assessment of the esophageal stage, including delayed esophageal transit time (<30 s is acceptable) and gastroesophageal regurgitation (Table 5.10).

5.3.1.1 Swallowing Study by VF: Anatomical Overview

Figures 5.9 and 5.10

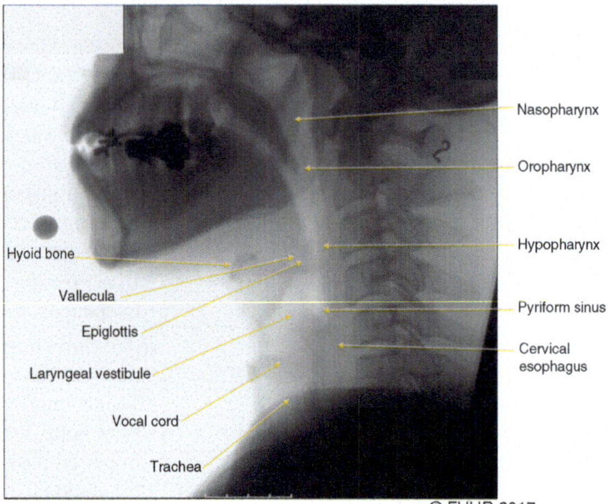

Fig. 5.9 Overview of oral and pharyngeal lateral fluoroscopic view

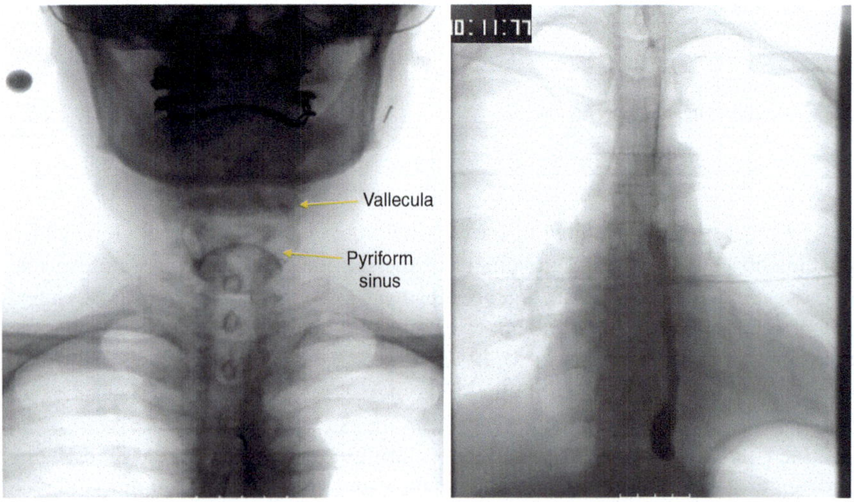

Fig. 5.10 Anteroposterior fluoroscopic images. (*Left*) overview of oral and pharyngeal view. (*Right*) esophageal view

5.3.1.2 Three Mandatory Evaluation Points During VF

Position of the Bolus Head at Swallow Initiation

Figure 5.11

Aspiration and Penetration

Figures 5.12, 5.13, and 5.14

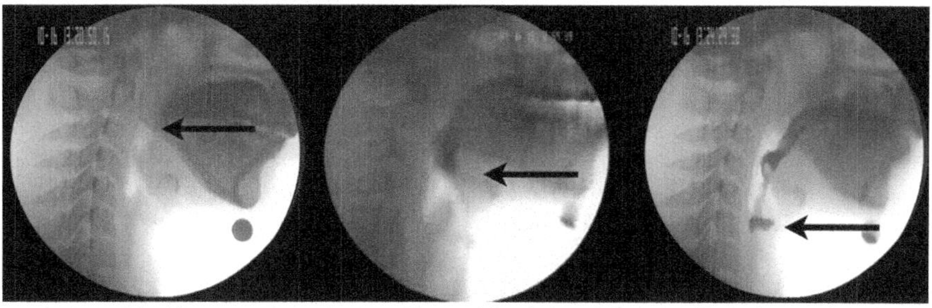

Fig. 5.11 Three leading edges of boluses. In a normal subject, the leading edges vary depending on the bolus type at swallowing onset, (*left*) liquid; swallowing onset occurs when the bolus head reaches the lower jaw line, (*middle*) corned beef; swallowing onset occurs when the bolus head reaches the vallecular, (*right*) two-phase food; swallowing onset occurs when some of the bolus reaches the lower area of the hypopharynx

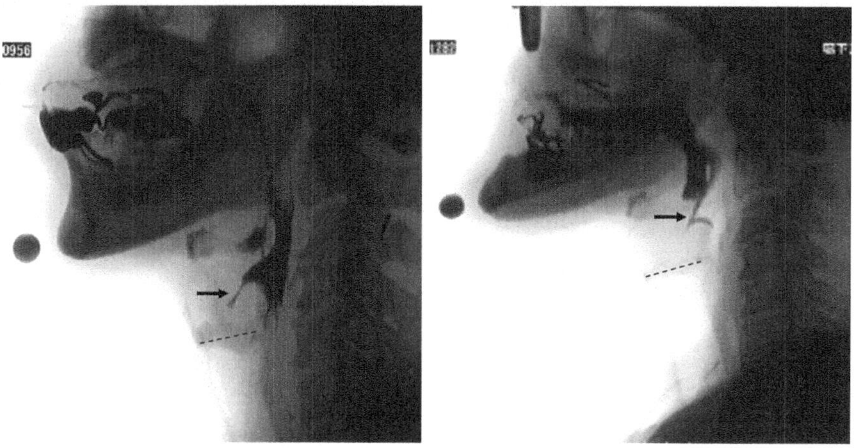

Fig. 5.12 Penetration (*arrow*) during swallowing on the lateral fluoroscopic view. The *dotted line* indicates the level of the true vocal cords

Determination of the cause of aspiration is the main purpose of a VF study, as shown in Table 5.11.

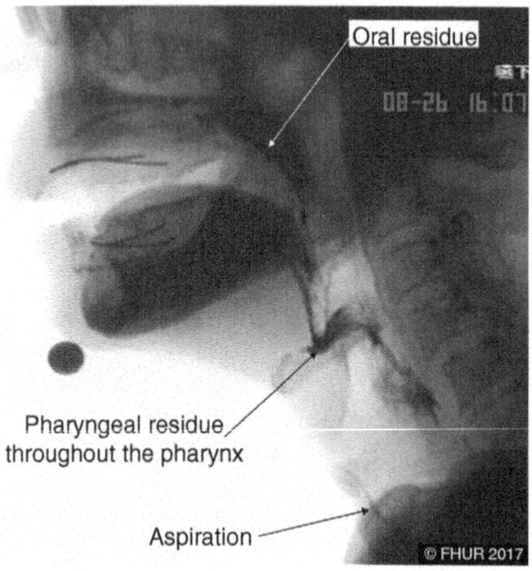

Fig. 5.13 Aspiration is demonstrated during a swallow on the lateral fluoroscopic view. The bolus enters the laryngeal vestibule down to the anterior wall of the trachea. Evidence of residue is present throughout the bolus pathway including the oral cavity, pharyngeal wall, vallecula, and pyriform sinus

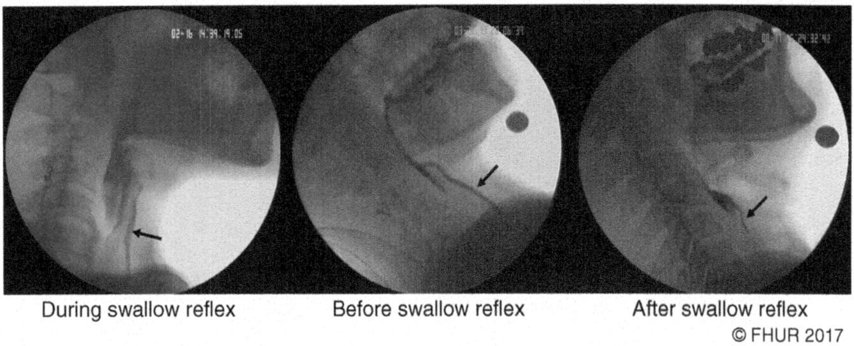

Fig. 5.14 Three types of aspiration (during, before, and after swallow), providing information regarding the patient's physiological abnormalities

Table 5.11 Possible causes of aspiration at three time points during videofluorography

Aspiration time	Possible causes
Aspiration *during* the swallow	Impaired laryngeal elevation
	Impaired laryngeal closure
Aspiration *before* swallow reflex triggered	Reduced tongue control, delayed or absent swallow reflex
Aspiration *after* the swallow (when the larynx lowers and opens for respiration)	Remained residue in the vallecula and pyriform sinuses from any reasons (such as weakened pharyngeal constrictors, reduced hyolaryngeal elevation, cricopharyngeal dysfunction), esophago-pharyngeal regurgitation

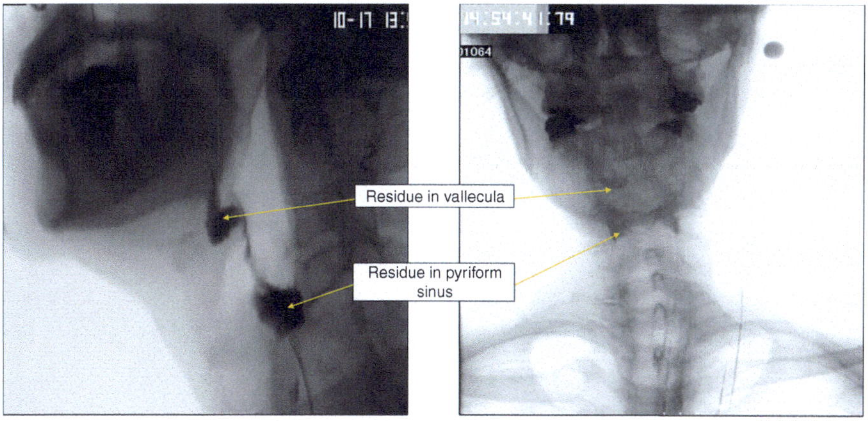

Fig. 5.15 Bolus residue at the vallecula and pyriform sinuses on the lateral and anteroposterior fluoroscopic views

Table 5.12 Possibly impaired mechanisms as predicted from the location of the residue

Location of residue	Impaired mechanism
Oral cavity	Incompetent bolus formation and propulsion (due to oromotor weakness)
Nasopharynx	Incompetent velopharyngeal closure
Tongue base	Inadequate lingual propulsion
Vallecula	Reduced/absent epiglottic retroflexion (due to reduce hyoid elevation), reduced base of tongue retraction
Pyriform sinus	Reduced pharyngeal shortening or reduced UES opening
Posterior pharyngeal wall	Reduced base of tongue retraction, weakened pharyngeal constrictors

Pharyngeal residue

Both the amount and location of the residue should be considered because this might allow the clinician to determine the risk of aspiration. The possibly impaired mechanisms may be identified from the location of the residue (Fig. 5.15; Table 5.12).

5.3.1.3 Other Abnormalities Identified by VF study

Figures 5.16 and 5.17

As previously described, VF is a treatment-oriented tool that can be used to determine the least difficulty task to provide swallowing rehabilitation training for prevention of aspiration while swallowing and reduction of the volume of residue in

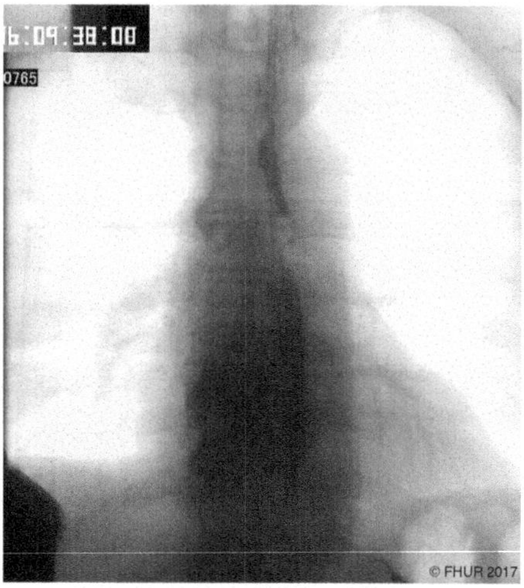

Fig. 5.16 Esophageal retention 30 s after swallowing caused by incompetent esophageal peristalsis; poor esophageal transit through the esophagus

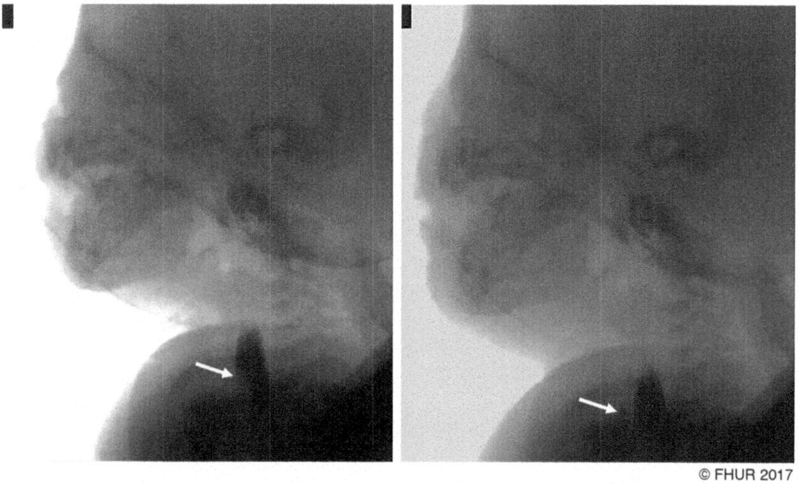

Fig. 5.17 Tracheoesophageal fistula is demonstrated during a swallow in an infant. The bolus passes into the laryngeal vestibule and enters the trachea

the pharynx. Aspiration and laryngeal penetration during VF can often be identified in dysphagic patients depending on various clinical variables. Essentially, VF can provide a clinical approach to enhancement of the safety of swallowing by changing the position of the patient's head and/or trunk and modifying various food parameters including consistency and bolus volume. The applicability of these postural strategies and food modifications is described in Part III (Figs. 5.18, 5.19, 5.20, 5.21, and 5.22)

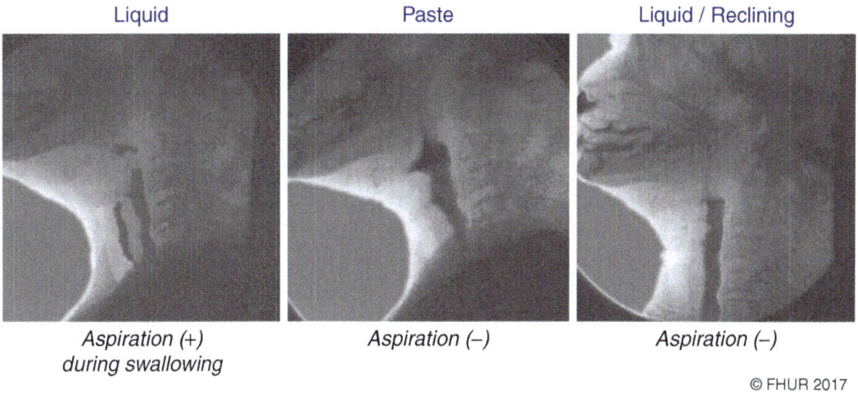

Fig. 5.18 VF provides an understanding of the least difficulty task that exists among these photographs. (*Left*) aspiration of liquid, (*middle*) modification of the food to become more paste-like can prevent aspiration, and (*right*) postural technique (reclining) to prevent aspiration during a liquid swallow. Thus, a safe exercise plan can be prescribed with combinations of these postures and food modifications

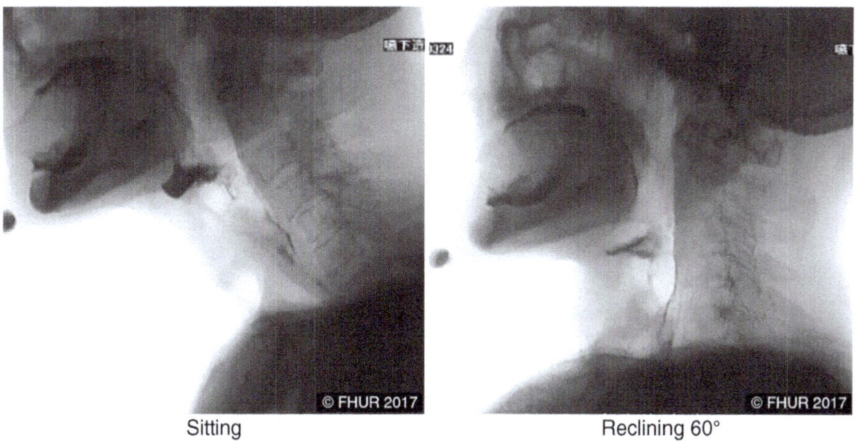

Fig. 5.19 Effect of the reclining posture during VF with a spoonful of rice porridge. (*Left*) sitting position; a large amount of residue is present in the oral cavity and vallecula after swallowing. (*Right*) reclining 60°; a decreased amount of residue is present in both the oral cavity and vallecula, and the time required for the swallow has been shortened

These factors should be included in each VF study to determine the most effective way to ensure safe swallowing. This will allow the clinician to recommend techniques to avoid aspiration, especially in patients with a high risk of silent aspiration.

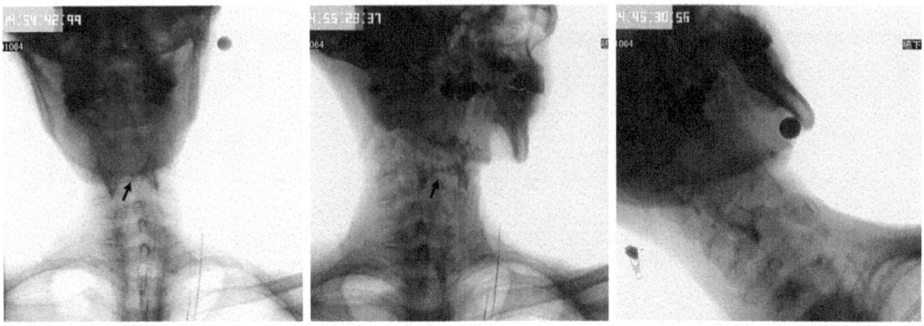

Fig. 5.20 Effect of trunk rotation with opposite head rotation to prevent aspiration during VF with a 2-mL bolus of nectar-thickened liquid (*arrow* = aspiration). (*Left*) neutral head position; a large amount of residue is present at the bilateral pyriform sinuses after swallowing, and aspiration has occurred after the swallow because of the residue in the pyriform sinuses and insufficient laryngeal closure. (*Middle*) left head rotation helps to reduce residue accumulation because of stronger pharyngeal contraction on the right side. However, head rotation alone is not enough to protect against post-swallowing aspiration. (*Right*) left head rotation with right trunk rotation; no signs of aspiration are seen even with a small amount of residue remaining

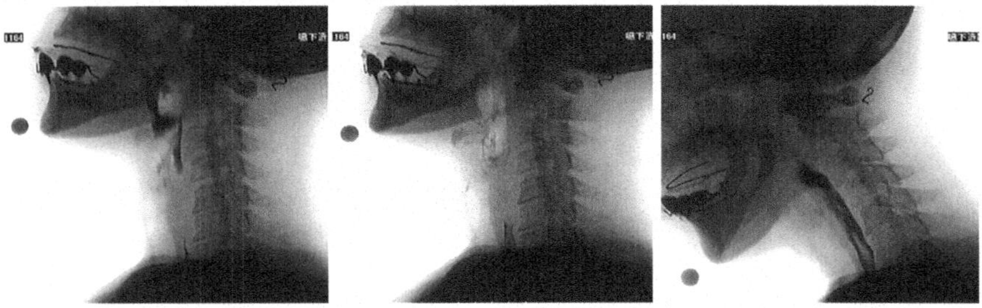

Fig. 5.21 Effect of head and neck flexion to prevent aspiration during VF with a 4-mL bolus of thin liquid

5.3.1.4 Analyses, Interpretation, and Reporting

The medical review of committee of JSDR published a manual for the standard VF procedure in 2001. VF evaluation forms and detail instructions regarding scoring are available in this manual. Analysis of the VF study results at FHUR is performed using the FHUR-VF evaluation form, which was originally made mostly based on the recent manual of the standard VF procedure [19]. Eighteen components are

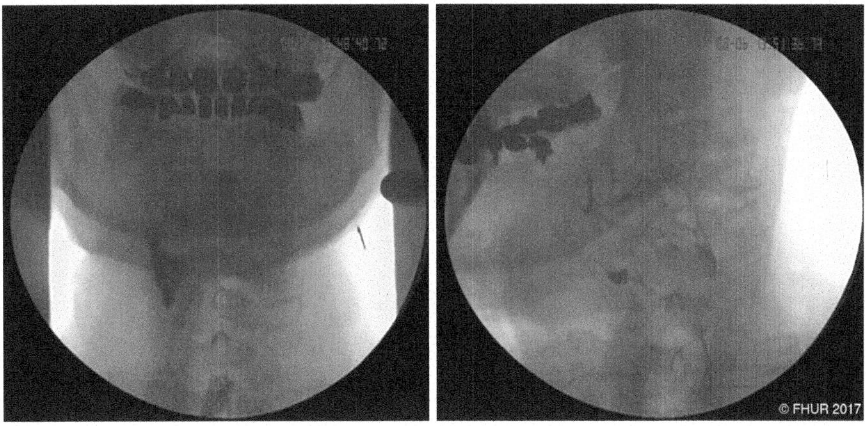

Fig. 5.22 (*Left*) a patient with Wallenberg syndrome. Bolus residue is present in the right pyriform sinus. (*Right*) right head rotation manipulates the space for changing the path of bolus flow in the pharynx and helps to minimize bolus residue in the right pyriform sinus, leading to a decreased risk of aspiration

evaluated, six in the oral domain, ten in the pharyngeal domain, and two in the esophageal domain (Fig. 5.23). Additionally, the eight-point Penetration-Aspiration Scale is used to evaluate aspiration. This scale provides reliable quantification of penetration and aspiration events during VF study [20]. The Penetration-Aspiration Scale is well known and has become the standard tool with which to describe the severity of penetration/aspiration. The scale is divided into eight different levels, and any score of >2 is considered abnormal (Table 5.13).

To summarize the results of each VF study, the SLHT scores every component for each bolus trial while performing the VF study. The DSS and ESS are used to rate the patient's functional swallowing problems and conditional eating status as well as guide the future treatment plan (Table 5.14) and recommendations regarding safe foods for the patient (Fig. 5.24).

Upon completion of the VF evaluation, the physiatrist, SLHT, and any other healthcare members involved in the investigation analyze all of the collected information.

The VF study report provides the following data:

1. Result of swallowing under all conditions used during the study
   - Lateral and anteroposterior views
   - Various volumes, consistencies, and textures of foods and liquids
   - Postural techniques and swallowing maneuvers
   - Behavior and compliance of patient
2. Nature of the swallowing problem: most likely pathophysiologic mechanism of swallowing impairment

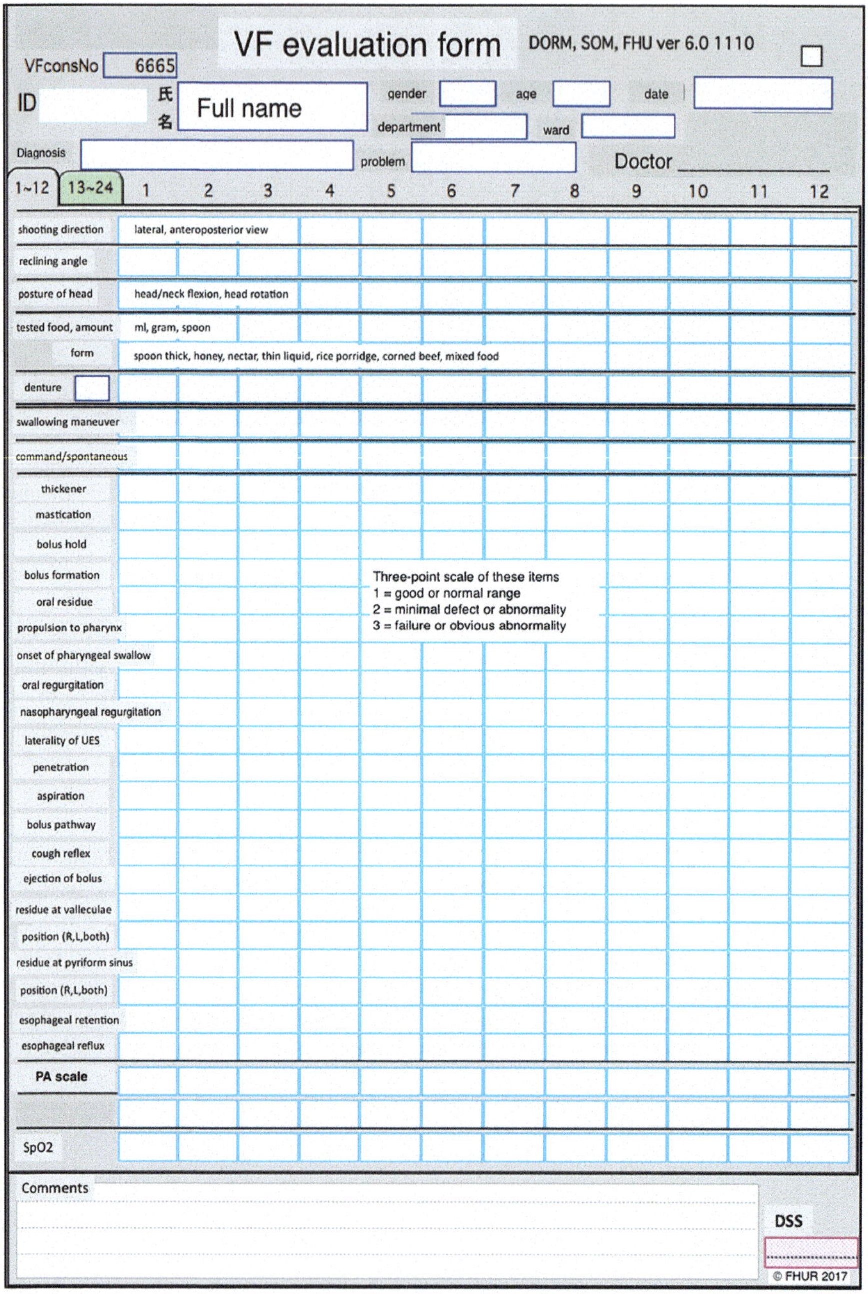

VF evaluation form DORM, SOM, FHU ver 6.0 1110

VFconsNo 6665

ID 氏名 Full name gender age date

department ward

Diagnosis problem Doctor

1~12 13~24

		1	2	3	4	5	6	7	8	9	10	11	12
shooting direction	lateral, anteroposterior view												
reclining angle													
posture of head	head/neck flexion, head rotation												
tested food, amount	ml, gram, spoon												
form	spoon thick, honey, nectar, thin liquid, rice porridge, corned beef, mixed food												
denture													
swallowing maneuver													
command/spontaneous													
thickener													
mastication													
bolus hold													
bolus formation													
oral residue													
propulsion to pharynx													
onset of pharyngeal swallow													
oral regurgitation													
nasopharyngeal regurgitation													
laterality of UES													
penetration													
aspiration													
bolus pathway													
cough reflex													
ejection of bolus													
residue at valleculae													
position (R,L,both)													
residue at pyriform sinus													
position (R,L,both)													
esophageal retention													
esophageal reflux													
PA scale													
SpO2													

Three-point scale of these items
1 = good or normal range
2 = minimal defect or abnormality
3 = failure or obvious abnormality

Comments

DSS

© FHUR 2017

Fig. 5.23 VF evaluation form used at FHUR (Modified and translated into English)

Table 5.13 Penetration-Aspiration Scale [20]

Score	Descriptions
1	Material does not enter the airway
2	Material enters the airway, remains above the vocal folds, and is ejected from the airway
3	Material enters the airway, remains above the vocal folds, and is not ejected from the airway
4	Material enters the airway, contacts the vocal folds, and is ejected from the airway
5	Material enters the airway, contacts the vocal folds, and is not ejected from the airway
6	Material enters the airway, passes below the vocal folds, and is ejected into the larynx or out of the airway
7	Material enters the airway, passes below the vocal folds, and is not ejected from the trachea despite effort
8	Material enters the airway and passes below the vocal folds, and no effort is made to eject

3. Timing (before, during, or after swallowing) and cause of aspiration
4. Decisions regarding the most appropriate treatment plan
   - Safest modified food and drink
   - Essential therapeutic interventions and exercises needed

5.3.1.5 Equipment

At FHUH, we use a digital X-ray television system (ZEXIRA DREX-ZX80; Toshiba Medical Systems Corporation, Otawara, Japan) and a digital video recorder (WVD9000; SONY, Tokyo, Japan). The fluoroscopy system typically consists of a radiograph detector, radiograph source (X-ray tube), and a monitor and is located in the examination room. The X-ray is converted into video images that can be recorded for further evaluation and analysis. The ability to record the studies using the highest possible number of images generated per second is essential for accurate interpretation and analysis. The optimal frame rate is ≥30 frames per second captured on a recording system. This frame rate is used in our center and is a practical recommendation to prevent the clinician from missing significant pathology. A VF study chair (Tomei Brace Co., Ltd., Seto, Japan), the reclining level of which can be adjusted based on the patient's ability, is used during the examination.

5.3.1.6 Oral Contrast Media for VF study

The test material used during VF is important. To view a bolus under fluoroscopy, all foods and drinks must contain a radiopaque portion for visualization of the dynamic movement of the swallow under fluoroscopy. No gold standard technique of preparing contrast media for VF has been established. The most recommended

Table 5.14 Dysphagia severity scale: functional Dysphagia Severity Scale and recommended treatment plan

Level		Definition	Explanation	Intervention	Direct exercise
No Aspiration	7: Normal	No clinical problem	Treatment unnecessary	Unnecessary	Unnecessary
	6: Mild problem	Mild problem including subjective complaints	Various problems including major complaints that impact the patient's eating and swallowing ability	Interventions such as simple exercise, food modification, and denture adjustment are performed as necessary	Performed as necessary
	5: Oral problem	No aspiration, but problem with oral preparatory and/or oral propulsive stage	Main problem involves the oral stage, including the anticipatory and oral preparatory stage, increasing the risk of dehydration and malnutrition	*Exercise, modified food recommendation, and adjustment of eating under supervision based on oral function evaluation	Performed either in general healthcare center or at home

Aspiration	4: Occasional aspiration	Occasional aspiration or marked accumulation of residue that may cause aspiration	Marked pharyngeal residue or occasional aspiration during VF; suspected aspiration during meal	**In addition to (*), evaluation of and intervention to improve pharyngeal function and impact of mastication	Performed either in general healthcare center or at home
	3: Water aspiration	Aspiration with thin liquid but not with modified food/liquid	Aspiration of thin liquid with no response to special technique to eliminate aspiration and residue; food modification is still sufficient to prevent aspiration	In addition to (**), intermittent tube feeding should be considered for liquid intake	Performed either in general healthcare center or at home
	2: Food aspiration	Aspiration of almost everything without respiratory problem	Aspiration of all kinds of food (thin, semisolid, and solid food) without positive response to food modification	Unable to tolerate oral feeding; parenteral/tube feeding is necessary	Performed only with swallowing professionals
	1: Saliva aspiration	Aspiration of everything including saliva with unstable respiratory status; poor respiratory condition because of no swallowing reflex	Unstable medical condition with saliva aspiration	Intervention for stable medical status is the primary issue, and parenteral/continuous tube feeding is necessary	Impossible

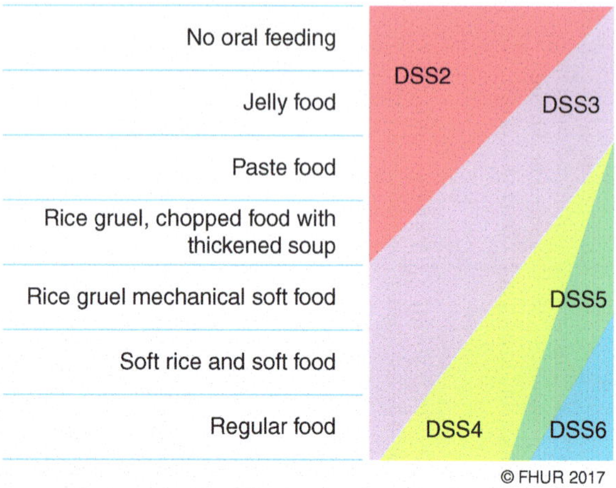

Fig. 5.24 Dysphagia Severity Scale score is used to recommend the most appropriate diet type for dysphagic patients (Recommended diet of DSS 2 is used merely in swallowing exercise with professionals)

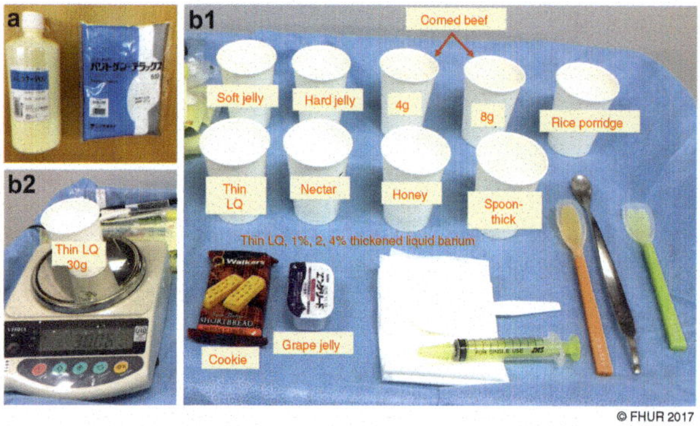

Fig. 5.25 (**a**) Liquid suspension and powder form of barium sulfate used at FHUR. (**b1**, **b2**) Equipment prepared for VF study

concentration for oropharyngeal swallowing examination is 40% weight/volume (W/V), which provides adequate visibility and prevents the clinician from missing critical events such as silent aspiration. Alteration of the barium concentration could influence the result of the evaluation. Thus, clinicians must carefully consider this issue when conducting and interpreting a VF study.

A barium sulfate formulation with a 100% W/V ratio (Bamstar S 100; KAIGEN, Osaka, Japan) is used to make an oral contrast media for VF study at FHUR. Foods and liquids with various viscosity, consistency, and texture are prepared according to our recipe. We dilute the barium sulfate suspension by 50% using water, and we then add a thickening powder to adjust the consistency as needed. The bolus materials prepared for VF in our institution are thin liquid barium, nectar-thickened liquid barium, honey-thickened liquid barium, spoon-thick liquid barium, corned beef hash (100 g/can of corned beef is mixed with 10 mL of 100% W/V barium suspension and 15 g of barium powder), rice porridge, soft and hard barium jelly, and cookie (Fig. 5.25; Tables 5.15 and 5.16).

Iodine-based, nonionic contrast medium (low osmolality) such as Iopamiron 300 (Bayer Japan, Tokyo, Japan) is recommended for VF in infants and young

Table 5.15 Summary of the properties of modified foods used for VF study at FHUR

Category	Bolus	Concentration of barium	Texture
Liquid	Thin liquid	50% W/V	16 mPa s
	Nectar-thickened liquid		140 mPa s
	Honey-thickened liquid		467 mPa s (50 s–1, 20°C)
Jelly	Soft jelly	40% W/V	Hardness, 1698 N/m^3; cohesiveness, 0.5; adhesiveness, 40.0 J/m^2
	Hard jelly		Hardness, 17280 N/m3; cohesiveness, 0.3; adhesiveness, 194.5 J/m^2
Semisolid	Rice porridge	Mixed with Ba	Hardness, 5120 N/m^3; cohesiveness, 0.7; adhesiveness, 1542 J/m^2
	Corned beef hash	Mixed with Ba	Hardness, 24,000 N/m^3; cohesiveness, 0.5; adhesiveness, 3570 J/m^2
Solid	Cookie	Coated with Ba	

Table 5.16 Sequence of boluses commonly used during VF study at FHUR

1. 4 mL of honey-thickened liquid barium
2. 4 mL of thin liquid barium
3. 10 mL of thin liquid barium
4. 8 g of corned beef hash
5. Two-phase food (mixture of 4 g corned beef hash and 5 mL of thin liquid barium)
6. Cup drinking (30 g) of thin liquid barium
7. Other test materials are used occasionally based on patient's condition

children and is used at FHUR. This contrast agent is a clear, colorless water solution with sufficient efficacy to provide images. It is commonly used to visualize vessels but can also be used for other purposes (e.g., intrathecally, intra-abdominally, and for cystourethrography). The advantage of this contrast agent is that it is more easily absorbed and less irritating to tissues when leakage into the tissues occurs. Additionally, it is less likely to cause pulmonary edema or fluid shifts in patients if they had occured aspiration of contrast agent into the lungs during VF. Because of its high cost, this agent is predominantly utilized in infants and young children. A number of pediatric studies have revealed that this lower-osmolality contrast agent is well-tolerated by infants, including medically fragile patients, during gastrointestinal tract examinations.

5.3.1.7 Performance of VF study

The setup for a VF study using a special swallowing chair and the positioning required for lateral projection are shown in Fig. 5.26. The patient's posture can be adjusted based on his or her history and condition. The patient is initially placed in

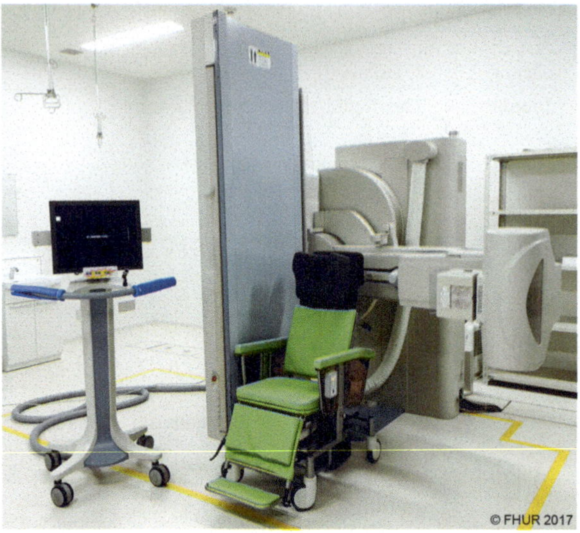

Fig. 5.26 Fluoroscopy suite prepared for swallowing examination using a special swallowing chair and positioning required for lateral projection

the lateral position to obtain an overview of the entire swallowing process. The oxygen saturation and heart rate are monitored in every patient during VF. A suction system is prepared as necessary.

In 1999, the Fujita Swallowing Team developed a special swallowing chair for VF study ("VF style" chair; Tomei Brace Co., Ltd.). The third and most recent modification was released in 2014. This model was designed for multifunctional use with an emphasis on more convenience. It acts like a multifunctional electric chair and has the following features (Fig. 5.27):

1. The chair is compact and smooth. It can be used in the limited space of a radiographic room. This chair also provides casters which rotate in multiple directions and is therefore easily moved the position from lateral view to the A-P view during the VF study.
2. The posture of the chair is easy to adjust during the VF study. Both a reclining angle and sitting height can be used, and these changes are made with an electric remote control to shorten the adjustment time.
3. The chair is stable and comfortable; it provides a headrest, leg rest, and foot rest as well as a brake locking system.

5.3.1.8 Radiation Safety

Many studies have confirmed that the effective dose of radiation associated with VF studies is safe [21–23]. One study in our center determined the amount of fluorescence after X-ray exposure during VF based on a 5-min interval, which is the standard time required for VF from both the lateral and A-P views [24]. The maximum exposed dose absorbed through the skin was 25.30 milligray (mGy)

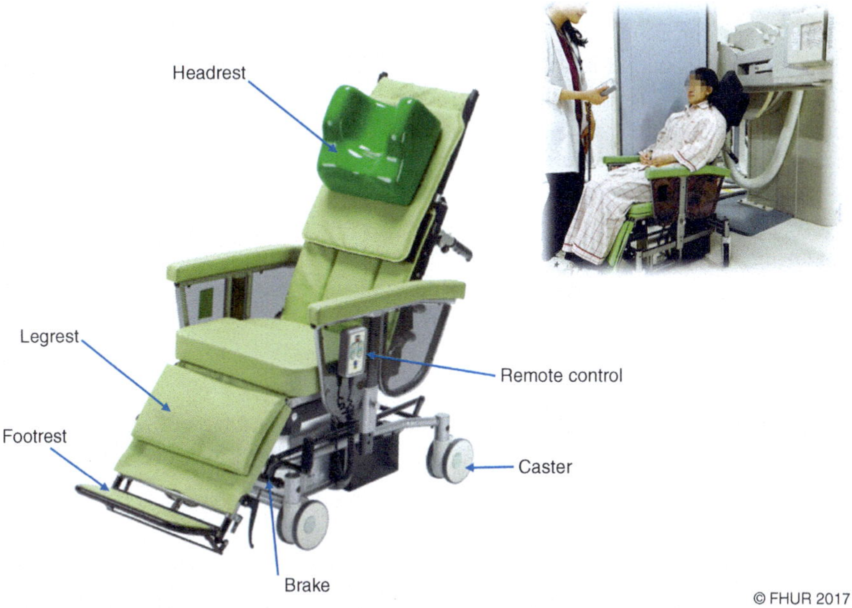

Fig. 5.27 Multifunction electric chair for VF study

(1.05 millisievert, mSv), which was smaller than the threshold value of 2000 mGy for early adverse skin effects (transient erythema). This means that VF can be performed using minimal radiation doses within a safe range and that the level of detrimental radiation associated with VF is acceptable.

5.3.2 Swallowing Examination by Videoendoscopy (VE)

Like VF, swallowing examination using VE has been proposed as a gold standard assessment technique. VE allows for treatment-oriented evaluation of swallowing function, enabling the patient to achieve a safe swallow and the clinician to formulate an effective treatment plan based on the patient's swallowing ability. It has relatively low invasiveness, is well-tolerated, is low-cost, and has the advantage of portability, allowing it to be easily and quickly performed at the bedside without radiation exposure.

VE is performed with the use of a flexible laryngoscope placed into the nose and extending down to the pharynx to view the pharyngeal and laryngeal structures during swallowing. VE permits a static and dynamic evaluation of the structures in the upper airways and upper digestive tract. It allows for easy, direct visualization of the pharynx during swallowing and the ability to gain information regarding pathophysiological deficits of the palate, pharynx, and larynx.

VE provides direct views of the surface anatomy, mucosal abnormalities, effects of altered structures on bolus flow and airway protection, vocal cord closure, bolus path, and bolus location in the hypopharynx. This technique also exhibits pooling of secretions, bolus formation and movement, and the patient's ability to swallow various bolus textures and consistencies. VE has therefore become a useful assessment tool with which to identify salient findings and guide treatment planning.

Figures 5.28 and 5.29 illustrate the anatomic structures viewed with VE.

During the performance of VE, three main observational points must be carefully considered for a thorough anatomic-physiologic assessment (Table 5.17; Fig. 5.30).

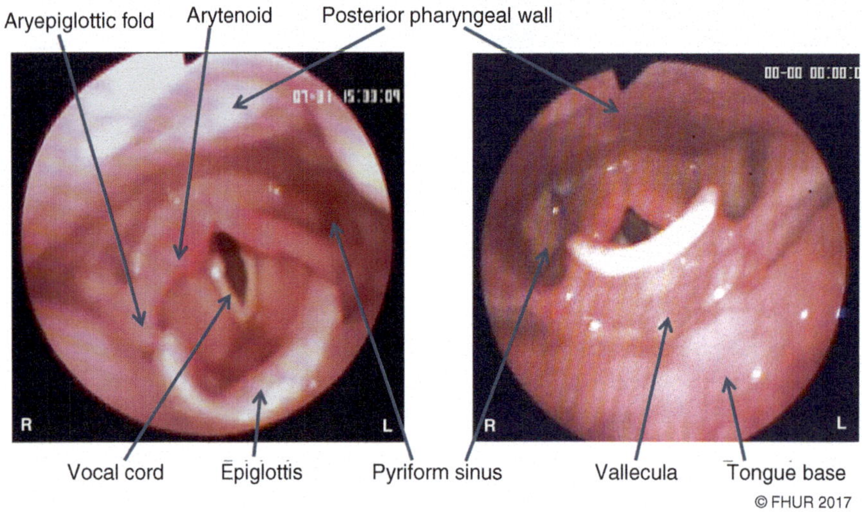

Fig. 5.28 Anatomic structures viewed with the endoscope placed within the oropharynx and hypopharynx (home position)

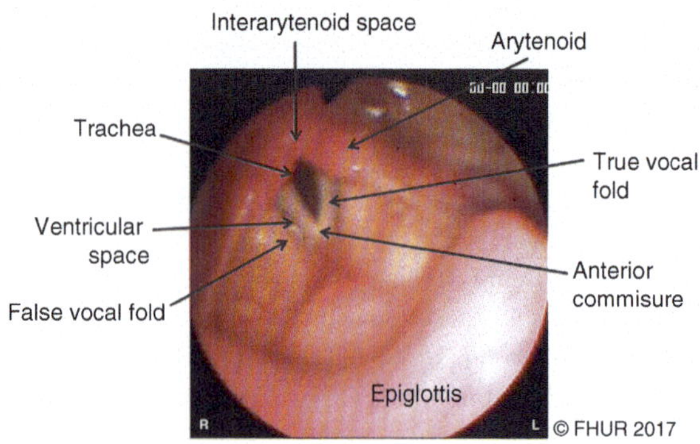

Fig. 5.29 Close view of laryngeal structures as seen with the endoscope

Table 5.17 Three main observational views during VE study

View no.	Location area	Key lookings
First	Nasopharynx	Soft palate, Lateral and posterior pharyngeal walls
Second	Oropharynx	Overview: secretion status
		Structures: tongue base, posterior pharyngeal wall, vallecula, pyriform sinuses
Third	Hypopharynx or laryngopharynx (posterior to epiglottis)	Vocal cords, arytenoids, pyriform sinuses

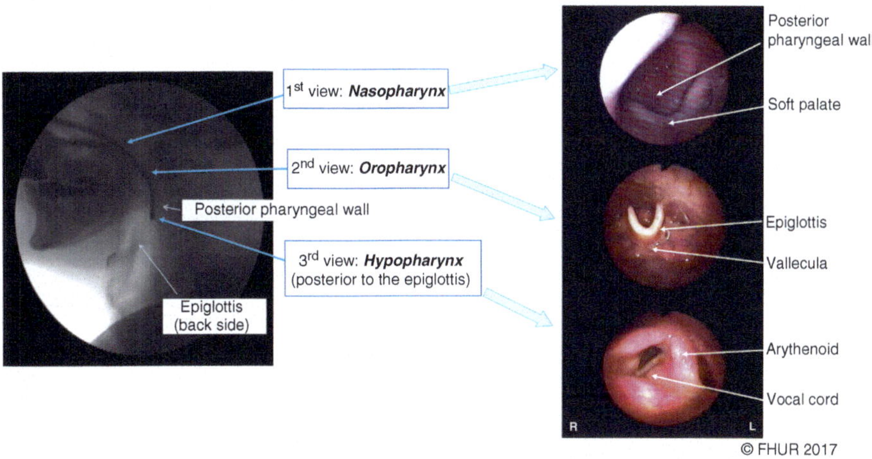

Fig. 5.30 Comparison of three main observational views between VE and VF

5.3.2.1 First View: Nasopharynx

The main target of the first view is functional evaluation of the nasopharyngeal structures, including soft palate elevation and nasopharyngeal muscle contraction. During vocalization and swallowing, VE allows for visualization of velopharyngeal closure upon contraction of the upper lateral pharyngeal walls and elevation of the soft palate, and both sides can be equally viewed. Thus, velopharyngeal insufficiency or saliva/bolus reflux can be observed in this view (Figs. 5.31, 5.32, and 5.33).

5.3.2.2 Second View: Oropharynx

This view is the pre-swallow position (high position, home position). The tip of the endoscope is maintained between the soft palate and tip of the epiglottis, where the entire larynx and recesses are visualized as shown in Fig. 5.28.

VE captures several structures that can be used to identify anatomical abnormalities at rest, including signs of inflammation (redness, edema), tumors, and

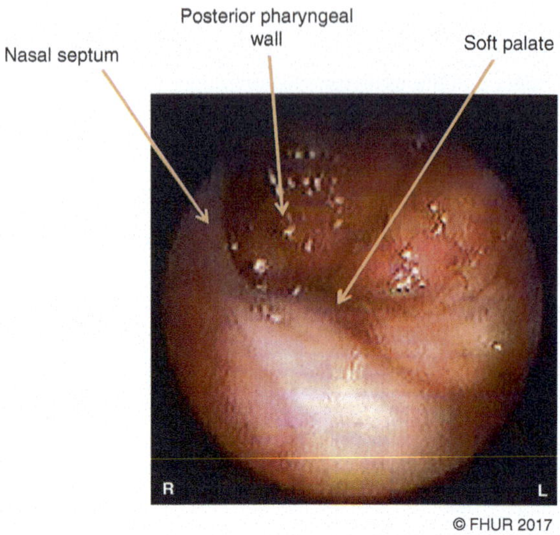

Fig. 5.31 Nasopharyngeal view. The laryngoscope is inserted transnasally through the inferior nasal meatus

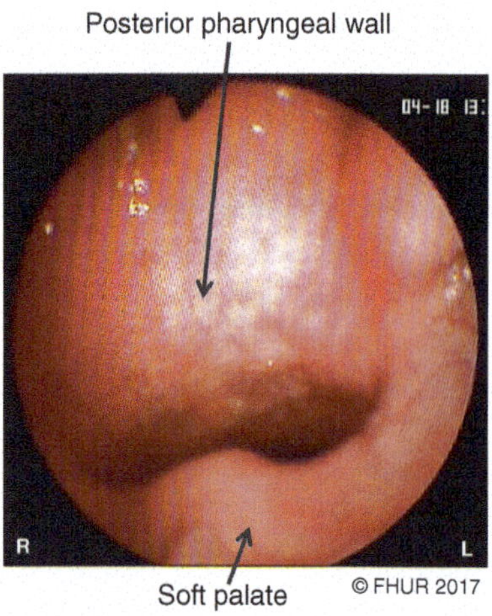

Fig. 5.32 View after tip of the endoscope has been advanced to the nasopharyngeal area

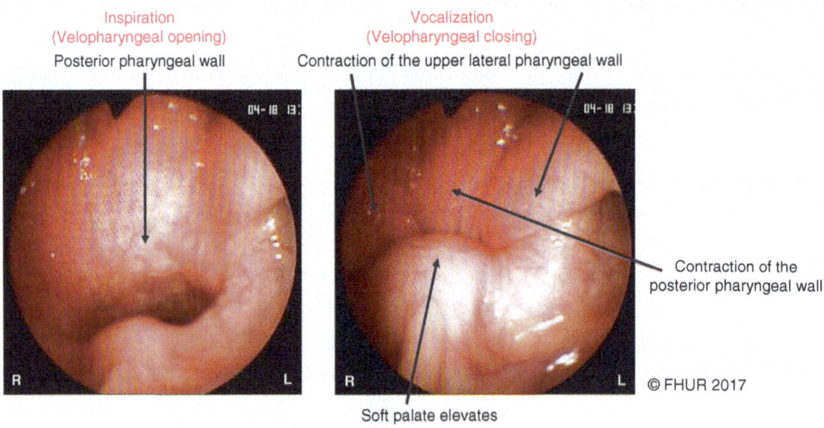

Fig. 5.33 Velopharyngeal closure during vocalization

the properties of the mucous membrane (pale, dry). It is important to evaluate the presence of pharyngeal and/or laryngeal secretion as well as the amount and location of accumulation. Tongue base movement while testing the bolus flow of various foods and liquids can also be observed in this view.

The bolus formation ability, especially with food that requires chewing, is an extra examination point in VE that provides useful information. Additionally, the position of the bolus head at the onset of the swallowing response can be directly inspected in the oropharyngeal view. This visualized position allows for optimum identification of premature spillage of a bolus and delayed pharyngeal response to the bolus.

5.3.2.3 Third View: Hypopharynx or Laryngopharynx (Posterior to the Epiglottis)

This view is a low position. The endoscope is directed along the posterior pharyngeal wall and reaches behind the epiglottis. The arytenoids, projections of the corniculate and cuneiform cartilages, aryepiglottic folds, true and false vocal cords, and ventricles are well visualized in this position (Fig. 5.29). Slight rotation of the endoscope in this position will clearly reveal the pyriform sinuses.

With a view of the hypopharynx, the endoscopy captures the onset of tongue retraction, epiglottal retroflexion, and lateral pharyngeal wall contraction during swallowing (so-called white-out, during which the scope is positioned against the posterior wall, while light reflects into the objective lens). When approaching the larynx, the endoscope allows for direct visualization of laryngeal closure, which includes both airway protection and the anterior wall of the trachea. Laryngeal closure involves the arytenoid approaching to the base of the epiglottis, vocal cord adduction, and backward folding of the epiglottis to cover the arytenoids and glottis. The occurrence of penetration or aspiration is also determined from this point of view, which shows whether bolus material or saliva has fallen into the subglottic region (Figs. 5.34 and 5.35).

5.3.2.4 VE Procedure at FHUR

The VE study and important findings obtained from the VE study are explained below. All VE studies are video-recorded for further analysis.

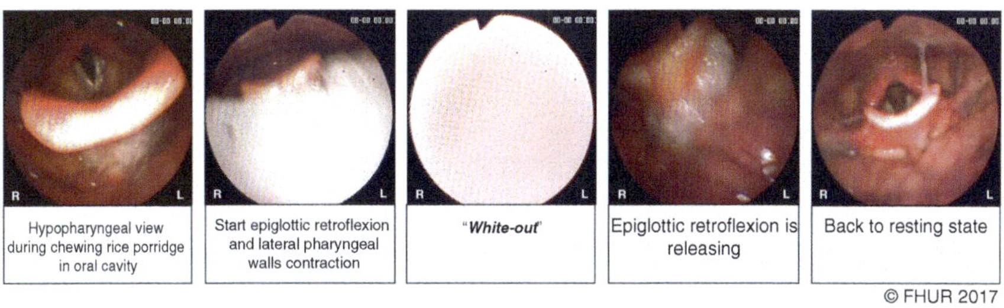

Fig. 5.34 Events before and after white-out

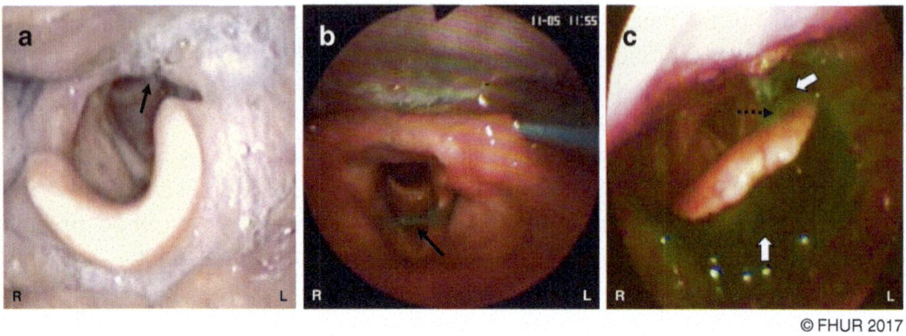

Fig. 5.35 (**a**) Aspiration of saliva, (**b**) aspiration during the swallow, and (**c**) penetration with a large amount of residue in the vallecula and left pyriform sinus

Evaluation Before the Use of Bolus Materials

1. The anatomy and function of the oral cavity are assessed.
   - Tongue movement (up–down, left–right, licking around lips), tongue deviation
   - Oral hygiene inside the oral cavity, the presence of oral residue or secretions
   - Soft palate elevation during phonation of "Ah" (symmetrical or asymmetrical)
2. Lubricant gel is applied to the distal part of the laryngoscope, avoiding contact with the tip of the scope (objective lens).
3. The laryngoscope is slowly and gently passed through the nasal cavity while avoiding contact with the nasal wall until the scope reaches the nasopharyngeal area.
4. The patient is instructed to phonate "ka" three times and then swallow saliva (dry swallow). The movement of the posterior pharyngeal wall, lateral pharyngeal walls, and soft palate elevation (velopharyngeal closure) is carefully observed.
5. The tip of the endoscope is advanced to a position between the soft palate and the tip of the epiglottis (behind the level of the uvula; "high position"). This position allows for visualization of the pharyngeal cavity and larynx at rest. The pharyngeal cavity includes the vallecula, base of the tongue, posterior pharyngeal wall, lateral pharyngeal walls, pyriform sinuses, epiglottis, arytenoid cartilages, and laryngeal inlet. Bolus transit in the oral preparatory/propulsive stage prior to swallow initiation is also easily observed in this view.
6. The hypopharyngeal space is observed. The presence, amount, and location of saliva, secretions, and residue are noted, especially in the vallecula space, pyriform sinuses, laryngeal vestibule, and trachea. If secretion is present, the ability of the patient to manage the secretion and swallow will be assessed by coughing and then swallowing.
7. The endoscope is advanced to a position closer to the larynx ("low position"). Anatomical abnormalities of the larynx and laryngeal vestibule, such as polyps, cysts, or edema, are observed. The functional movement of the true vocal folds (glottic closure) during phonation of "ee" is observed. The patient is asked to perform this phonation repeatedly to check the symmetry and precision of glottic movement (Fig. 5.36).

8. The patient is instructed to hold his or her breath lightly (for inspection of closure of the true vocal folds) and very tightly (for inspection of the ventricular folds and arytenoids) and then cough for evaluation of airway protection (laryngeal closure). The patient is also instructed to hold his or her breath for a few seconds to determine whether the duration of the maintenance of laryngeal closure during the pharyngeal swallow is sufficient (Fig. 5.37).
9. The patient is asked to perform a dry swallow for observation of pharyngeal constriction. This causes the light from the tip of the laryngoscope of reflect off of the tissue apposition (so-called white-out). This occurs in approximately half a second in normal subjects and prevents visualization of the pharynx bolus during swallowing.
10. Examination is performed with the use of bolus materials.

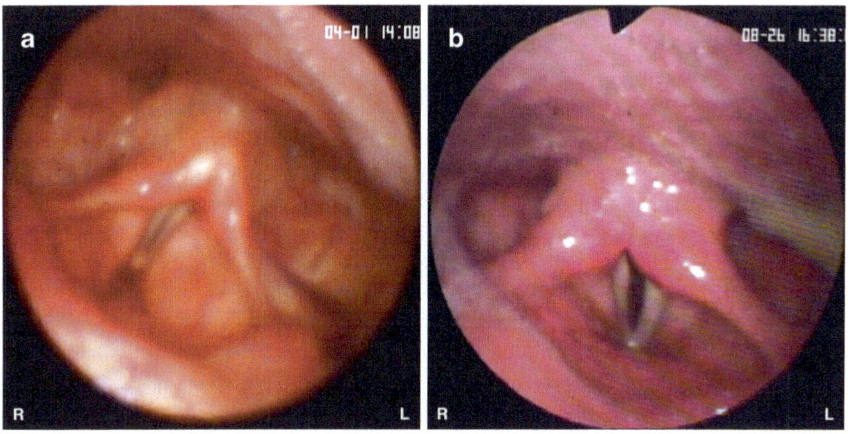

Fig. 5.36 (**a**) Normal glottis closure, (**b**) left recurrent laryngeal nerve palsy (left vocal cord paralysis)

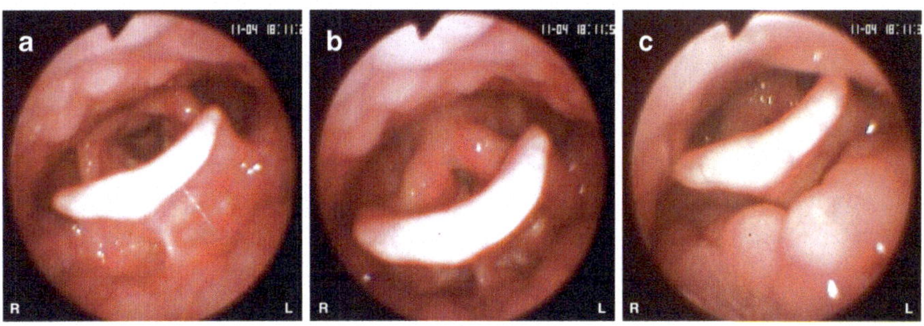

Fig. 5.37 (**a**) Normal breathing, (**b**) holding breathing lightly (closure of true vocal folds), and (**c**) holding breath tightly (closure of all laryngeal structures)

Evaluation with the Use of Bolus Materials

1. At the "high position," the swallowing reflex (pharyngeal response) is observed after the patient is instructed to swallow or chew–swallow; the bolus progression and bolus formation, particularly during the chew–swallow, are also observed. During the swallowing reflex, a white-out image is formed due to tissue apposition.
2. After the white-out period, bolus retention in the valleculae and pyriform sinuses is observed, and the endoscope is rapidly advanced into the area of the laryngeal vestibule to check for penetration (the bolus enters the laryngeal vestibule but is still above the level of the true vocal folds) and aspiration (the bolus enters the subglottic region).
3. At certain times, bolus aspiration may create an endoscopic blind spot at the posterior wall of the subglottic airway. If aspiration is suspected, the clinician should ask the patient to cough and monitor ejection of the bolus from the subglottic area. Changes in the voice quality, such as the development of a gurgling voice, should also be evaluated.
4. Various bolus volumes, consistencies, and textures should be used to clarify the patient's swallowing function. The VE study also allows the clinician to determine the effects of various combinations of postural strategies and swallowing maneuvers on pharyngeal residue and aspiration.
5. The safest and most appropriate foods, drinks, exercises, and treatment strategies for the patient are determined.

The VE promotes determination of the difficulty level of tasks, serving as a treatment-oriented tool, used in swallowing rehabilitation training (food modification and postural strategies) to prevent aspiration and eliminate residue in the pharynx (Tables 5.18).

While administering the VE study, the examiner should primarily focus on the bolus formation ability, timing of swallowing onset (delayed/absent), aspiration/penetration before or after swallowing, bolus clearance ability, and location and amount of residue. The types of food boluses and order of food testing are individually determined. The safest bolus food is always used first, and the difficulty of the swallow test is gradually increased. The level causing aspiration/residue should be detected to determine the patient's swallowing ability. The efficacy of therapeutic strategies (repetitive swallow, effortful swallow, etc.) and postural changes (neck or head flexion, head rotation, etc.) should be evaluated to find the strategy to eliminate aspiration and/or residue.

During the VE study, the patients and/or caregivers can observe the swallow on the monitor screen. Real-time visual biofeedback allows them to view and understand the swallowing ability, including the effectiveness of therapeutic strategies. This is helpful in enhancing patient compliance during dysphagia rehabilitation and ensuring successful outcomes.

However, VE does have some limitations. It does not enable visualization of certain critical aspects of the pharyngeal swallow (e.g., tongue base retraction, level

Table 5.18 Important issues that must be examined during VE

Part 1: before bolus testing
1. Oral mechanism examination • Movement of the tongue, soft palate • Oral hygiene, oral residue or secretion, denture
2. Overall appearance of the oropharynx, hypopharynx, and larynx • Anatomical abnormalities: edema, erythema, excrescences (nodule, lump, cyst), evidence of reflux
3. Secretions • Patient's tolerance • Dry swallow initiated • Characteristics of secretion (thick, clear, yellow, bubbly)
4. Function • Velopharyngeal closure (competence) • Base of tongue retraction • Sensation for swallowing initiation • Pharyngeal contraction • Laryngeal closure (epiglottis retroflexion, complete and symmetrical closure of bilateral true vocal cords, medicalization and forward tilting of bilateral arytenoids)
Part 2: while bolus testing
Monitor path of bolus at two points: 1. Pre-swallow position (oropharynx) 2. Post-swallow position (hypopharynx)
1. Mastication • Duration, the property of bolus formation in vallecula
2. Premature spillage, delayed pharyngeal response
3. Penetration (deep, shallow)/aspiration
4. Residue • Amount, location, patient's response

of airway closure, UES opening). Additionally, the oral and esophageal stages of the swallow (e.g., chewing ability, esophageal transit, gastroesophageal regurgitation) cannot be assessed well. There is also a temporarily blocked view (white-out) from the endoscope during laryngeal elevation while swallowing; this may cause the clinician to miss an aspiration event such as that resulting from a bolus located at the posterior wall of the trachea. In these cases, VF is more likely to reveal problems (Table 5.19).

5.3.2.5 Equipment

Figures 5.38 and 5.39

In our facility, we prepare several types of foods and liquids for VE study as shown in Fig. 5.40. Blue- or green-dyed food and liquid materials of various volumes and consistencies are used during the VE study to enhance the bolus visualization.

Table 5.19 Common indications for VE and VF

Characteristics	VF	VE
Oral stage dysfunction	✓	
UES dysfunction[a]	✓	
Esophageal stage dysfunction	✓	
The effectiveness of compensatory strategies and maneuvers	✓	
Hyolaryngeal excursion	✓	
Laryngeal penetration and aspiration[b]	✓	✓
Pharyngeal residue	✓	✓
Delayed swallowing response	✓	✓
Poor oral hygiene/oral residue		✓
Secretion and saliva aspiration		✓
Direct visualization of laryngeal structure		✓
Real food/liquid evaluation		✓
ICU patient/bedside evaluation (portable)		✓

[a]*UES* upper esophageal sphincter
[b]Except aspiration during swallowing reflex can be detected only by VF

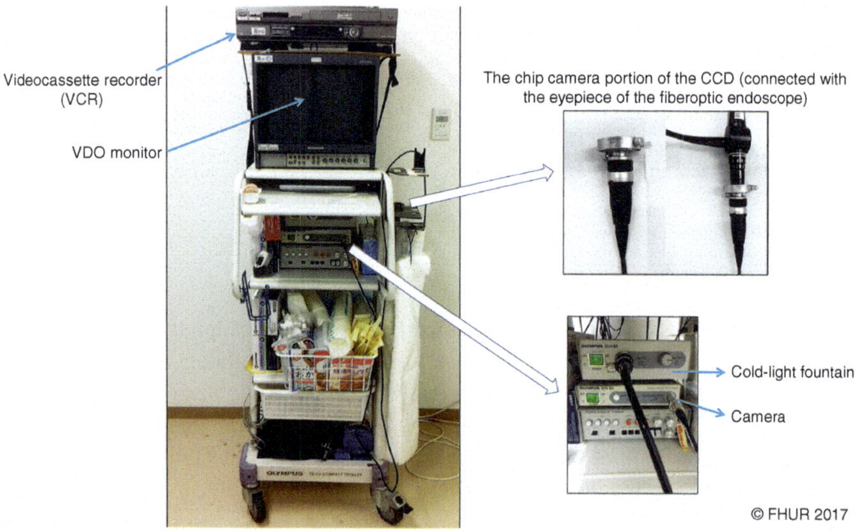

Fig. 5.38 Portable endoscopy unit used during VE study

5.3.2.6 Performance of VE study

Before performing VE, clinicians should have adequate knowledge of the anatomical structures around the nasal and pharyngeal cavity, pharynx, and larynx.

The patient either sits or reclines depending on his or her medical condition. A flexible endoscope is placed transnasally through either the inferior nasal meatus

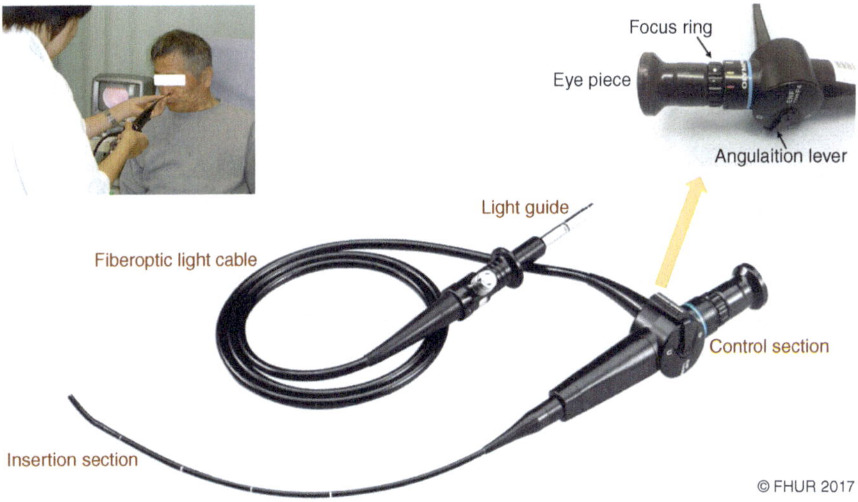

Fig. 5.39 Configuration of basic flexible laryngoscope

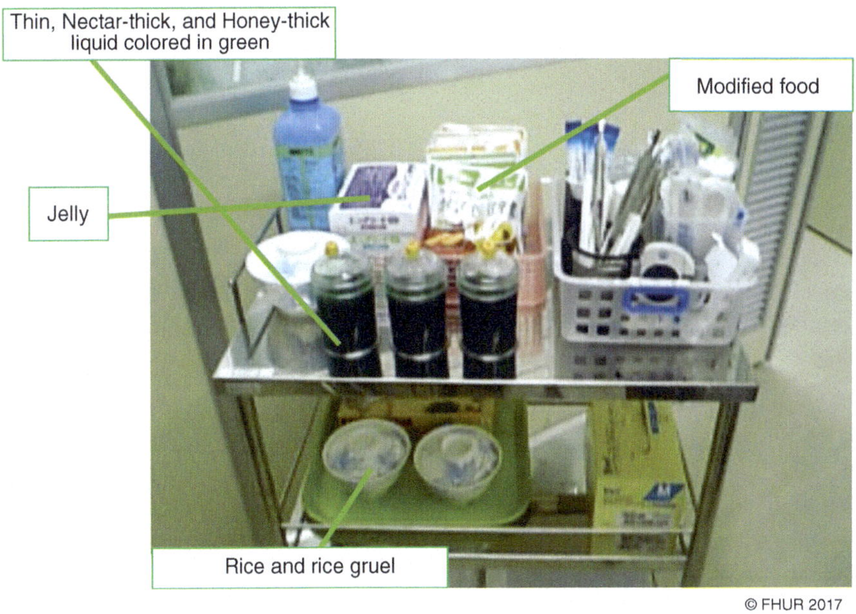

Fig. 5.40 Bolus materials prepared for VE study

(lowest nasal passage between the inferior nasal concha and nasal floor) or middle nasal meatus (space between the middle nasal concha and inferior nasal concha) (Fig. 5.41). The flexible laryngoscope is advanced to the nasopharynx until it reaches the position at which the clinician attains a holistic view of the oropharynx. The

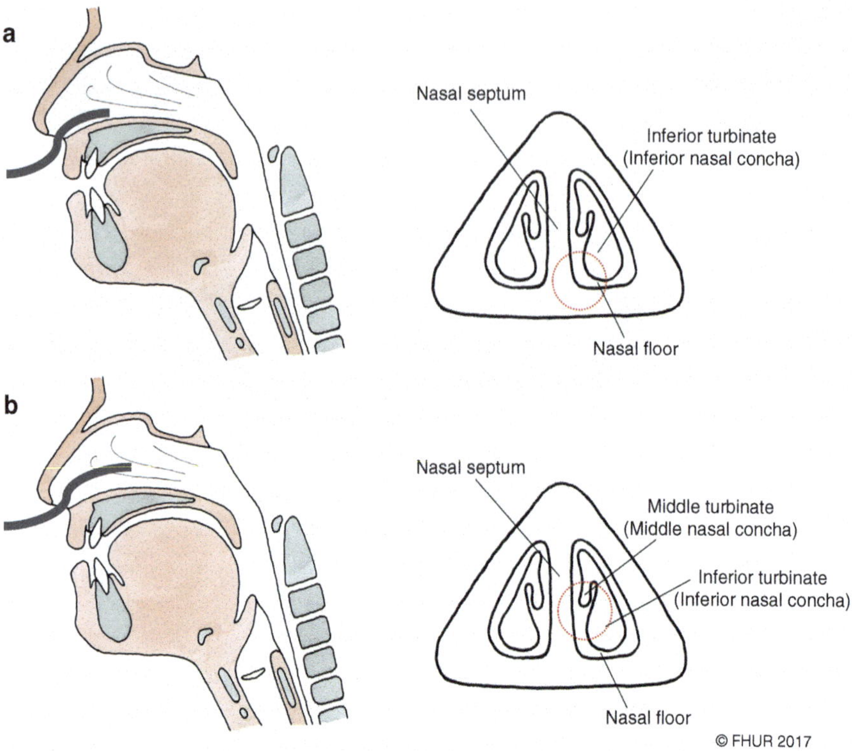

Fig. 5.41 Insertion of endoscope through the nostril (**a**) via the inferior nasal meatus and (**b**) via the middle nasal meatus

clinician can visualize the image directly through the eyepiece or by using a camera attached to the laryngoscope, which shows the image on a video monitor. The video in connection with the recording of results is also available for further analysis.

5.3.2.7 Examination Safety

VE is a safe and effective swallowing evaluation method. The overall rate of complications associated with VE is <1% [25]. Moreover, none of these complications are serious. Most patients cooperate and tolerate the VE study well [26]. The potential risks associated with VE include nasal bleeding, vasovagal syncope, laryngospasm, and gagging [25, 27]. A previous study revealed that only three (<1%) cases of nasal bleeding occurred among 500 flexible endoscopic evaluations of swallowing with sensory testing and there was no evidence of laryngospasm, vasovagal response, or airway compromise [28]. Likewise, in 2009, a prospective study of the safety of flexible endoscopic evaluation of swallowing in patients with acute stroke demonstrated that nasal bleeding is the most prevalent VE-associated complication. However, all events were mild in severity and required no treatment, and all of the patients were able to continue the VE procedure [29].

5.3.3 *Systematic Evaluation in an Acute-Care Hospital (FHUR): Swallowing Ward Rounds with VE*

FHUR utilizes a highly efficient team structure for all dysphagic patients and conducts systematic evaluations using VE or VF after screening tests. These instrumental measures are therapeutically oriented examinations that allow for the diagnosis and evaluation of dysphagia and establishment of a plan for dysphagia rehabilitation.

Figure 5.42 illustrates the procedure for swallowing ward rounds (SWR) at FHUR. After a certified nurse of dysphagia nursing screens patients to determine who will require detailed investigations, the dysphagia care team conducts the SWR and evaluates patients by VE. The FHUR dysphagia care team comprises a physiatrist, dentist, SLHT, certified nurse of dysphagia nursing, nurse in charge of dysphagia in the ward, dental hygienist, and dietician. After diagnosis and evaluation of dysphagia, the treatment plan (including appropriate food, posture, oral care, and both direct and indirect training methods) and need for referral for further investigation by VF are determined as necessary (Fig. 5.43). All patients are followed up by the SLHT or certified nurse of dysphagia nursing even no intensive treatment is needed. During this follow-up, the patient's condition is monitored, and the treatment efficacy is determined. The certified nurse of dysphagia nursing can request reevaluation by VE as necessary.

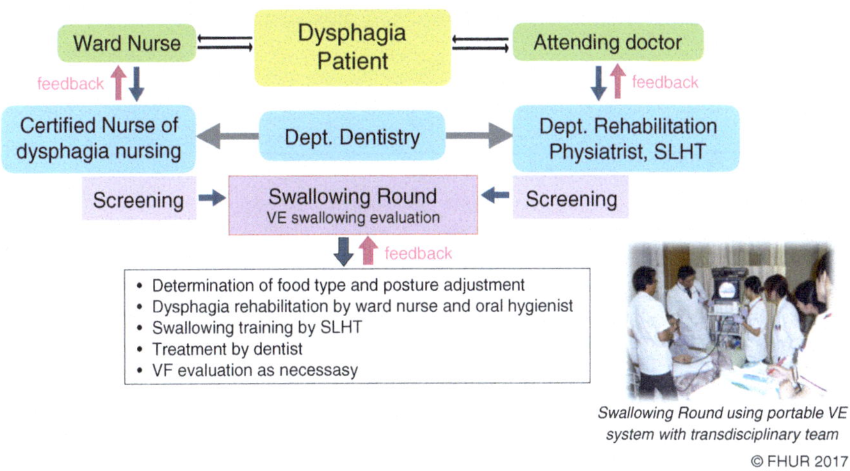

Fig. 5.42 System of swallowing ward rounds at FHUR

Videoendoscopy evaluation sheet

Name: operator:

Date: with/without tracheotomy: type with/without tubal feeding (R/L/cross)

Consciousness note SpO2: ⇨

Evaluation of Structure/function

Oral cavity hygiene: good/not (tongue coat/drying/bleeding/food residue)

Tongue motion: good/not laterality: +/– side of palsy: left/right

Soft palate phonation motion: good/not laterality: +/– side of palsy: left/right

swallowing motion: good/not laterality: +/– side of palsy: left/right

pharyngeal cavity tube: direct/cross/other left/right

hygiene: good/not bleeding +/–

salivary collection: not/small/moderate region: epiglottic vallecula/piriform recess/ interarytenoid fold/all

phonation wall motion laterality: +/– side of palsy: left/right

swallowing wall motion laterality: exist/not side of palsy: left/right

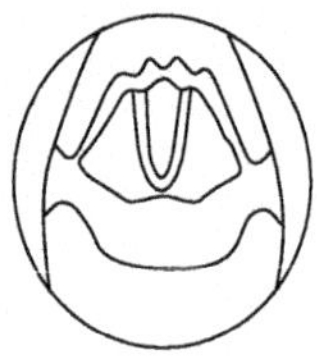

larynx vestibule salivary collection: exist/not aspiration: exist/not

arytenoid motion: good/not laterality: +/– side of palsy: left/right

vocal cord motion: good/not laterality: +/– side of palsy: left/right

white out: exist/not clear/not

type of food: comment

posture aspiration: not/small/moderate/unclear Expectoration: able/not/spontaneous/order

degree. sitting penetration: not/small/moderate Expectoration: able/not/spontaneous/order

head rotation: right/left residue: not/small/moderate Expectoration: able/not/spontaneous/order

type of food: comment

posture aspiration: not/small/moderate/unclear Expectoration: able/not/spontaneous/order

degree. sitting penetration: not/small/moderate Expectoration: able/not/spontaneous/order

head rotation: right/left residue: not/small/moderate Expectoration: able/not/spontaneous/order

type of food: comment

posture aspiration: not/small/moderate/unclear Expectoration: able/not/spontaneous/order

degree. sitting penetration: not/small/moderate Expectoration: able/not/spontaneous/order

head rotation: right/left residue: not/small/moderate Expectoration: able/not/spontaneous/order

RESULT: DSS: aspiration: apparent/occult request to dentist: need (denture/oral care/indirect exexcise)/not

Exercise ST: direct/indirect ( ) Dentist: oral care/indirect (functional therapy) ward: indirect/direct (functional therapy)

Feeding condition posture: G–up degree lateroversion/neck rotation

Morsal limitation/pasing/adding swallowing/alternate swallowing (thickened water gelly)/coughing

Food type: staple food: paste/gruel/soft rice/rice other food: paste/coarse paste/soft food & thickened water/soft food/rather soft food/normal

Water: 2.0%/1.5%/1.0%/liquid (spoon/spout cup/straw/cup)

Next evaluation: after W/ST order/after intake stable

Fig. 5.43 VE evaluation form used during swallowing ward rounds at FHUR (modified and translated to English)

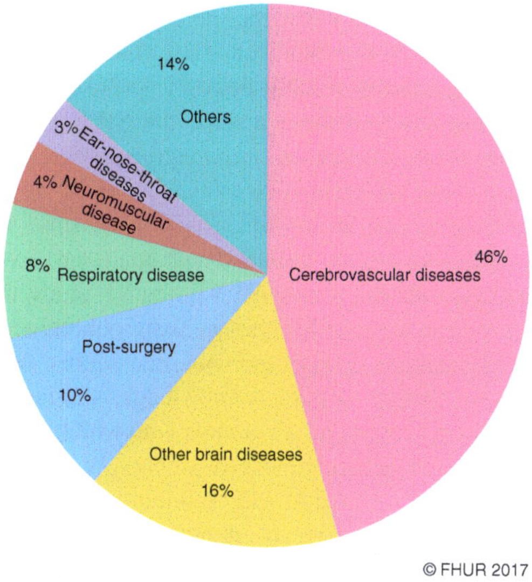

Fig. 5.44 Causes of dysphagia determined during swallowing ward rounds from 2006 to 2010 ($n = 998$); 455 (46%) patients had stroke, accounting for almost one-half of all patients

From September 2006 to March 2010, 1330 patients from the database of the FHUR dysphagia care team were identified and screened by a certified nurse of dysphagia nursing, and 998 of these patients were analyzed by SWR [30]. The most common causes of dysphagia were stroke (46%) and other cerebral diseases (16%) as shown in Fig. 5.44.

The patients' demographic characteristics are shown below.

- The average age was 74 years (range, 2–102 years).
- The median duration between admission and the first intervention was 13 days (range, 0–275 days).
- The median duration between the beginning and end of the first intervention was 24 days (range, 1–337 days).

After SWR using VE, proper treatment was selected from one of the following four groups:

1. Indirect or direct dysphagia rehabilitation performed by the SLHT.
2. Eating training performed by the SLHT and ward nurse.
3. Both 1 and 2.
4. Follow-up performed by the certified nurse of dysphagia nursing, who monitored the patient's condition after the clinician had prescribed the appropriate diet and posture. The ward nurses received advice regarding modifications of the food texture, postural adjustment, and training methods.

Treatment resulted in significant improvements in the food texture, ESS score, and DSS score between the first and last observations, indicating the effectiveness of SWR. Additionally, the incidence of pneumonia during the observation period (3.7%) was lower than that of one-third of patients in previous reports [31–33]. The implementation of SWR helped to prevent pneumonia.

According to these results, the SWR approach has the potential to facilitate appropriate evaluation and treatment of dysphagia, thus improving swallowing safety and efficiency. Notably, the SWR approach is particularly beneficial for evaluating swallowing function in the hospital setting.

Members of the FHUR dysphagia team have developed both a clinical practice and educational focus. All VE and VF study findings are reviewed and discussed weekly in an interdisciplinary team conference that includes a physiatrist, SLHT, certified nurse of dysphagia nursing, dentist, dental hygienist, and otolaryngologist. The exchange of pooled knowledge, sharing of ideas, and group discussion are important communication tools with which to improve the quality of teamwork and provide the best treatment to patients.

Moving forward, it will be important to promote scientific research that enables clinicians to gain a more comprehensive understanding of swallowing pathophysiology and contribute to the development of the best-practice methods for patients with dysphagia. Such research will both emphasize clinical inquiry and explore basic science. Thus, the FHUR dysphagia care team conducts a multidisciplinary research meeting once a month to disclose growth in this field of research and present the ongoing research by team members. These meetings enhance the interrelationship among practice, research, and education to advance the field of dysphagia for the ultimate benefit of the patient.

5.4 New Perspectives in Swallowing Assessment

Advances in technology over the past decade have enabled clinicians to use new and innovative tools to obtain more information about swallowing pathophysiology. All of the following techniques have been recently utilized for both research and clinical use at FHUR.

5.4.1 Swallowing Computed Tomography

Dynamic imaging tools (both VF and VE) are indispensable for standard treatment-oriented evaluation of dysphagia. They can be used to detect the risk of aspiration and presence of residue and determine the effectiveness of bolus modification and therapeutic strategies such as postural adjustments and swallowing maneuvers to eliminate aspiration and residue. Although VE and VF contribute to the understanding of swallowing pathophysiology, visualization of three-dimensional (3D) complex movement is limited. Thus, some mechanisms of swallowing physiology are incompletely understood.

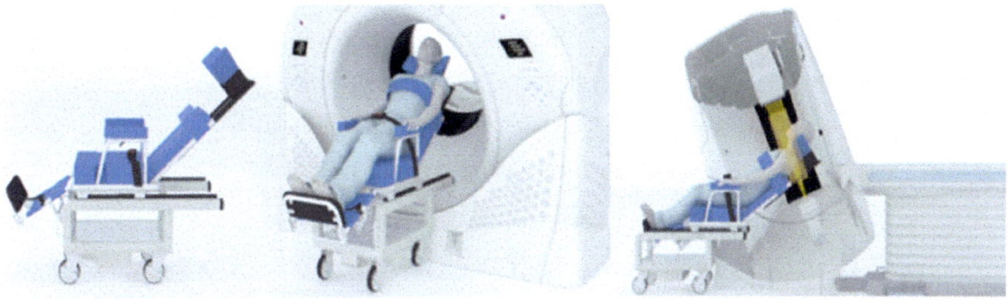

Fig. 5.45 Swallowing 320-ADCT with dedicated offset-sliding chair and scanning posture at the time of the CT

Dynamic swallowing computed tomography (CT), namely, 320-row area detector CT (320-ADCT) (Aquilion ONE; Toshiba Medical Systems Corporation), was developed and introduced in 2007 at FHUR to overcome this limitation (Fig. 5.45). This swallowing CT technique provided the first 3D visualization of swallowing worldwide. It revolutionized the whole-swallow examination and provided new insights into swallowing morphology and kinematics from two primary viewpoints: 3D dynamic imaging and quantitative measures. The dynamic movements of all swallowing structures throughout the swallowing process can be simultaneously evaluated from all directions, allowing for a highly accurate quantitative analysis.

5.4.1.1 Equipment and Performance

The 320-ADCT is equipped with 320 rows of 0.5-mm detectors along the body axis. It can acquire a volume data set covering a maximum range of 16 cm in one 0.275-s revolution with a non-helical scan. A 16-cm range can cover the area from the skull base to the upper esophagus, which is required for a complete swallowing analysis. Scanning is performed with the 320-ADCT system using a chair designed exclusively for the swallowing CT examination (eMedical Tokyo Co., Ltd., Chuo-ku, Japan; Tomei Brace Co., Ltd., Seto, Japan). The reclining CT chair is an offset-sliding chair that is fixed on a base and designed to slide forward and backward. The CT scanner is tilted to 22°. The reclining CT chair is placed on the opposite side of the CT table. The patient is seated on the chair in a semi-sitting position at 45°, and the chair is then slid backward into the middle portion of the scanning plane (Fig. 5.45).

5.4.1.2 Analysis and Clinical Utility

The CT images are reconstituted to 10 frames/s by the half-reconstruction method to create multiplanar reconstruction (MPR) images and 3D-CT images [34, 35]. MPR images allow for depicting structures on any arbitrary cross section in any orientation with 0.5-mm slice thickness and analyzing time and space quantitatively.

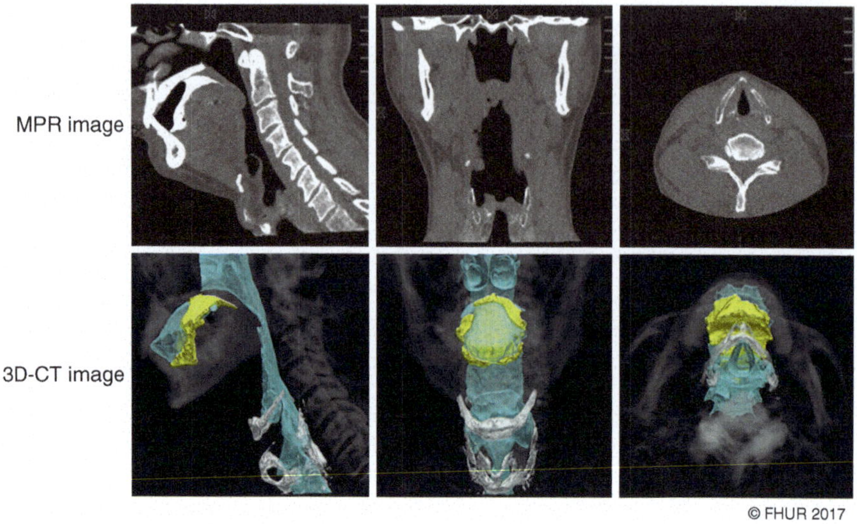

Fig. 5.46 MPR and 3D-CT images. (*Upper row*) MPR images: sagittal, coronal, and axial planes. (*Lower row*) 3D-CT images: lateral, posterior, and inferior views (the vocal cords can be visualized)

The 3D-CT images allow for visualization of the overall structural movements and performance of volumetric analysis (Fig. 5.46).

The outstanding property of several quantitative measurement tools facilitates a comprehensive understanding of both normal physiology and pathophysiological swallowing disorders in dysphagic patients. 3D-CT allows for several types of kinematic analyses of the temporal state (i.e., timing of structures' movement) and the spatial state (i.e., volume of pharyngeal residue or UES cross-sectional area). The following section of text describes the clinical availability of swallowing CT.

First, the 320-ADCT system is novel in that it allows the clinician to determine the opening/closing times of the vocal cords, which cannot be visualized using VF. The bolus consistency and volume influence the characteristics of swallowing, especially closure of the larynx. This information is very important for clarification of the airway protection system (Fig. 5.47).

Second, 320-ADCT allows for measurement of the onset and end of all structural movements that occur during the swallow. Measuring the times of all events is beneficial for kinematic analysis because it provides an understanding of the physiological mechanisms of swallowing, allows for comparison of the responses to diverse bolus types, and illustrates the pathophysiology of swallowing disorders compared with a healthy swallow (Fig. 5.48).

Third, dynamic measurement of the UES dilatational area is another unique benefit of swallowing CT. The UES can be identified with the landmark of thyroid cartilage and cricoid cartilage in the horizontal plane. The ability of 320-ADCT to capture dynamic cross-sectional images of the UES area during swallowing

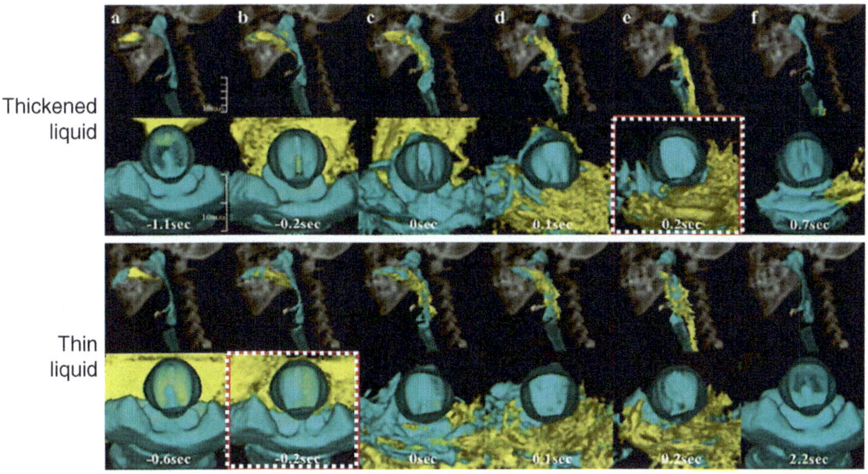

Fig. 5.47 Comparison of physiology between swallowing of thickened liquid and thin liquid. Closure of the vocal cords (*dot square*) occurred in the early stage when swallowing thin liquid (Reproduced from [36] with permission)

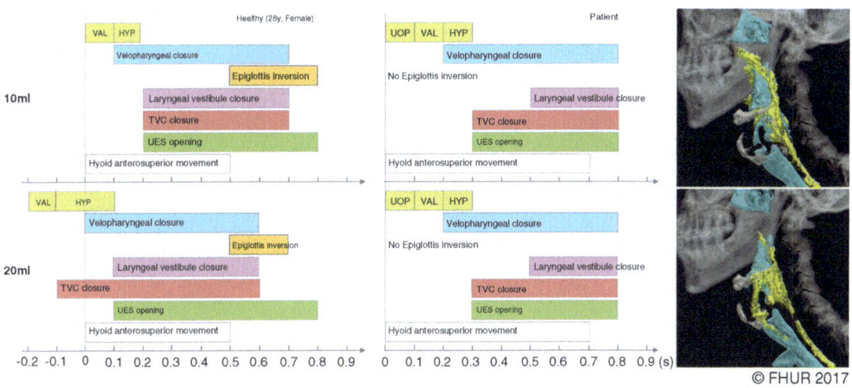

Fig. 5.48 Comparison of the whole process of swallowing 10-mL and 20-mL thin liquid boluses between a healthy subject and dysphagic patient (a 68-year-old man with dysphagia due to polyneuropathy). The figure shows the timing from the onset to end of the movements of various swallowing organs at the same time (*healthy subject*). The onset of hyolaryngeal movement and laryngeal closure is earlier when swallowing the larger bolus (*patient*). The onset of movement of all swallowing structures is delayed. The structural movement pattern generally shows no change with various bolus sizes. Failure of modification with an increased bolus size and the delayed onset of laryngeal closure elicit aspiration (Reproduced from [37] with permission)

facilitates an understanding of the relationships among hyolaryngeal excursion, UES opening, and pharyngeal residue accumulation (Fig. 5.49).

Fourth, during pharyngeal functional analysis, 320-ADCT provides excellent measurements of volume. It is possible to measure the volume of the pharynx during

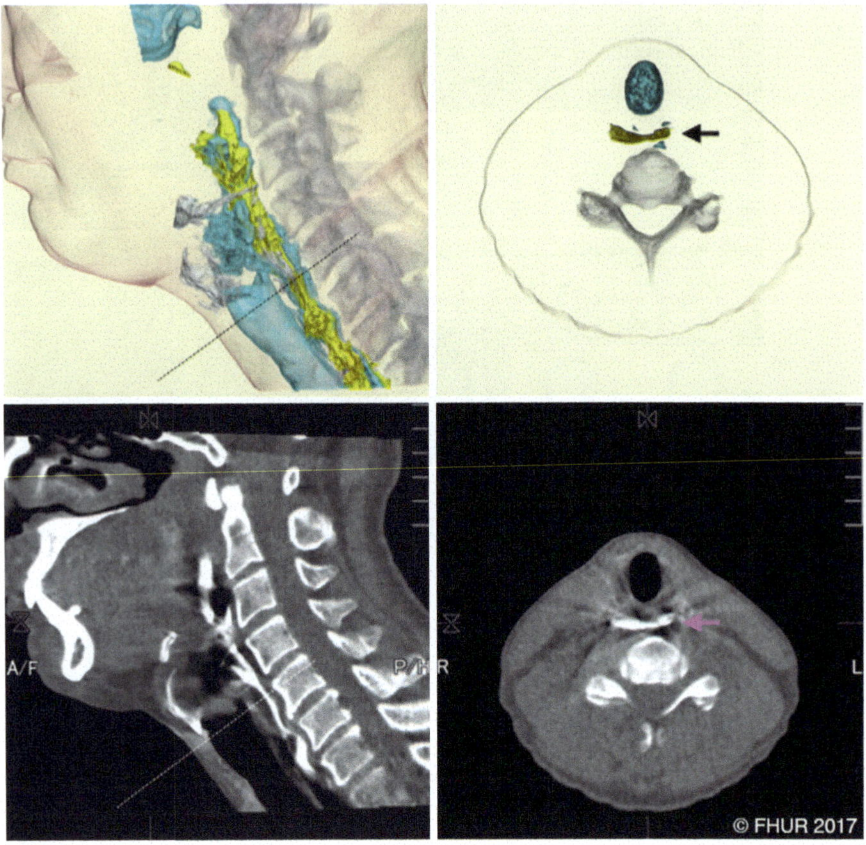

Fig. 5.49 Measurement of cross-sectional area of the UES during swallowing can be determined by 320-ADCT

the swallowing and to calculate the pharyngeal constriction ratio. It reflects the ability of pharyngeal contraction, promoting the analysis of pharyngeal residue accumulation (Fig. 5.50).

Finally, the dynamic motion of the hyoid and larynx during swallowing can be measured by analyzing the distance between the origin and insertion of swallowing muscles (length of the muscles) associated with the trajectory of these structures. Unlike VF, swallowing CT can be used to analyze the dynamics of the thyroid cartilage other than hyolaryngeal movement (Fig. 5.51).

One study showed that the average values of upward and forward movement of the hyoid bone were 16.5 ± 9.2 and 12.8 ± 5.0 mm, respectively. The study also revealed a significant correlation between shortening of the geniohyoid muscle and forward movement of the hyoid bone, whereas other suprahyoid muscles (including the stylohyoid, posterior digastric, and mylohyoid muscles) significantly contributed to upward movement of the hyoid bone [39].

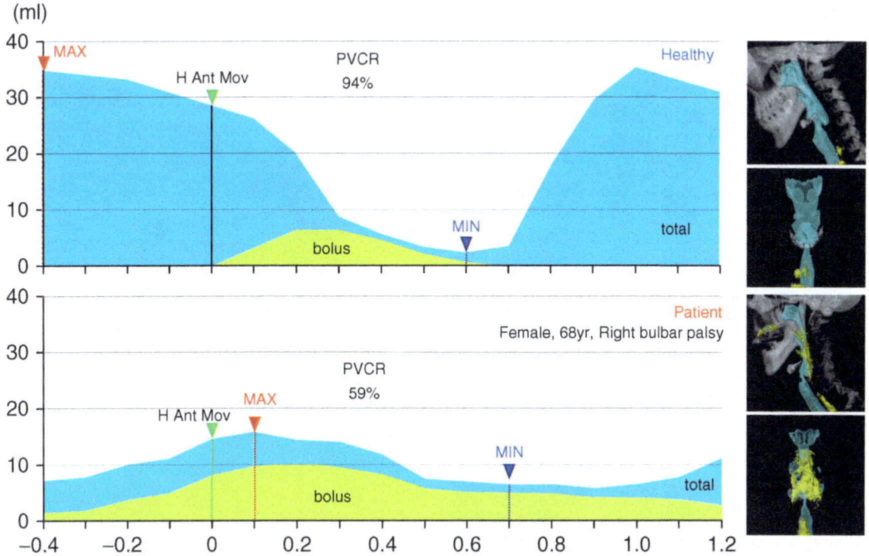

Fig. 5.50 Change in pharyngeal cavity during bolus swallowing. Patients with dysphagia show weakness of the pharyngeal constriction and a large amount of pharyngeal residue after swallowing. The pharyngeal cavity has changed little during swallowing, and the pharyngeal volume constriction ratio (PVCR) is nearly two times lower than that in a healthy subject. (*Upper*) a 34-year-old healthy woman. (*Lower*) a 68-year-old woman with dysphagia due to a right pontomedullary infarction (Reproduced from [38] with permission)

In addition to evaluation of the pathophysiological changes associated with swallowing disorders, 320-ADCT can be utilized to assess the outcomes of rehabilitation training programs and determine the effectiveness of swallowing strategies such as swallowing maneuvers [40] and postural strategies [41] with respect to swallowing mechanisms.

Thus, swallowing CT certainly serves as a useful treatment-oriented evaluation technique. Since it provided the first dynamic 3D images, swallowing CT has been successfully used to precisely visualize the dynamics of swallowing and has encouraged quantitative analysis. This has led to the development of more sophisticated, broader knowledge of swallowing. Swallowing CT is also becoming an indispensable tool for the innovation of new rehabilitative interventions and generation of deeply treatment-oriented evaluations to overcome the difficulty of tasks.

Nevertheless, 320-ADCT is not intended to replace VF; instead, it complements VF and allows the clinician to obtain more information while conducting a swallowing assessment. Swallowing 320-ADCT is thus a crucial tool that provides invaluable information in swallowing for both research and in the clinical setting. Such information will help in the establishment of new rehabilitation approaches.

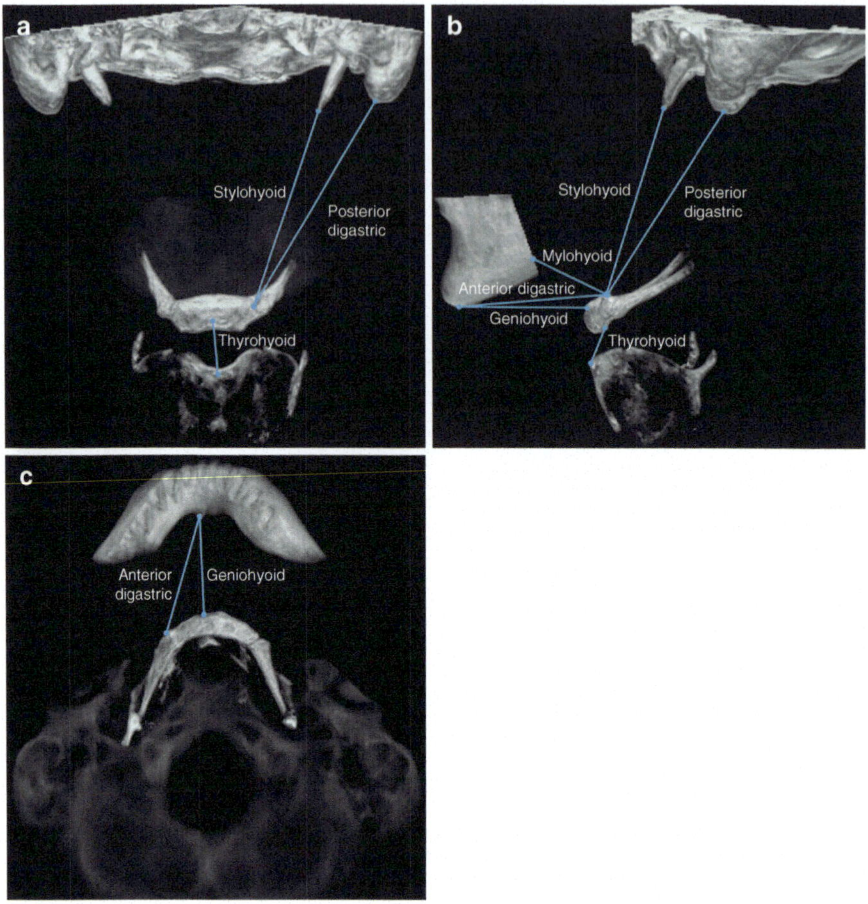

Fig. 5.51 Measurement of the distance between the origin and insertion of key swallowing muscles in three planes with the use of bony landmarks (mandible, hyoid bone, and thyroid cartilage), (**a**) anterior view, (**b**) lateral view, and (**c**) superior view (Reproduced from [39] with permission)

5.4.1.3 Examination Safety

With respect to the risk of radiation exposure during 320-ADCT (Aquilion ONE ViSION Edition, updated version of the original Aquilion ONE), the maximum dose absorbed through the skin is 28.07 mGy, which is smaller than the threshold level (2000 mGy) for detection of early transient skin erythema. The effective radiation dose for 320-ADCT is 1.08 mSv; this is lower than the 2.8-mSv dose required for a single neck CT scan, although it is still high compared with the effective radiation dose of a 5-min VF study [24].

5.4.2 High-Resolution Manometry

Quantitative movement analysis generally involves the acquisition of both kinematic and kinetic data. Combining both types of data is beneficial for obtaining a comprehensive understanding of swallowing physiology and advanced knowledge in a more purposeful way. As mentioned earlier, swallowing CT and VF are sophisticated techniques with which to perform kinematic analyses; however, kinetic data of the swallow, such as the pressure at the base of the tongue and pharyngeal constriction, are still lacking.

A new method called high-resolution manometry (HRM) was recently developed to obtain information on the pressure in the areas of the pharynx and UES during the swallow for a more complete understanding of swallowing pathophysiology.

The pharyngeal swallow is a complex pressure-driven process requiring intricate coordination of muscular contractions and pressure generation to efficiently move a bolus into the esophagus. While VF is the primary tool with which to obtain information on bolus transit, aspiration, and residue, it does not provide quantitative information on the changes in pharyngeal pressure underlying bolus transit and does not detect incomplete UES relaxation.

HRM can be used to directly measure the pressure along the pharyngeal area and provides quantifiably comprehensive data characterizing the real-time swallow. These data are recorded for subsequent analysis. Thus, HRM is useful for advancing the diagnosis and treatment of oropharyngeal dysphagia.

5.4.2.1 Equipment and Analysis

A typical HRM system includes a solid catheter with 36 circumferential sensors placed 1 cm apart to quantitatively measure pressure events (Fig. 5.52).

Pressure from the pharynx to the lower esophagus can be detected by passing and placing the catheter through the nose and into the esophagus. The result is displayed and analyzed in a spatiotemporal plot (so-called pressure tomography plot). The pressure tomography plot displays time on the X-axis and distance (position of sensor) on the Y-axis, and pressure values are coded by color. The result can also be illustrated with a line plot as shown in Fig. 5.53.

5.4.2.2 HRM Combined with VF or Swallowing CT

Although HRM is a useful tool for evaluation and analysis of contractile forces (pressure events) at the pharynx and UES, it alone cannot provide certain information that can be obtained from VF. HRM cannot be used to:

1. Accurately evaluate the pharyngeal response relative to the movement of the bolus

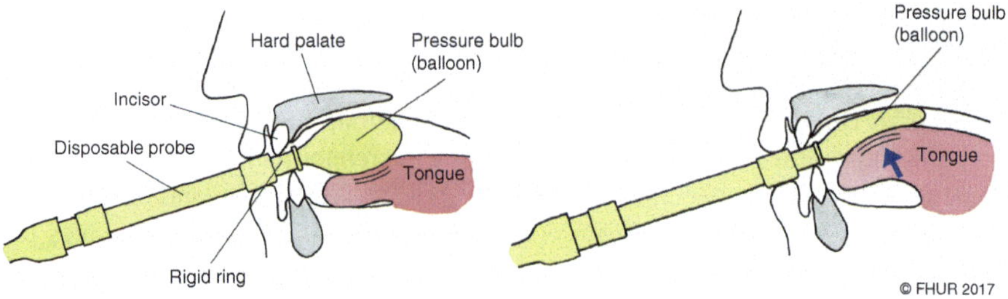

Fig. 5.57 Use of the tongue pressure measurement device

Our facility has also recently been researching tongue pressure measurement using another type of device: a sensor plate system. This device has four measuring sensors that detect the tongue pressure at four points. This allows us to focus on the local tongue strength at each point and compare both sides for symmetry. The mouthpiece of the sensor plate is directly attached to the hard palate, preventing the sensor from sliding on the tongue surface like the balloon-type pressure bulb and increasing the measurement accuracy.

Because of the important role of the tongue pressure in swallowing function, measurement of this parameter has high potential for clinical use, especially in patients with diseases or conditions associated with the development of tongue weakness such as stroke, Parkinson disease, and head and neck cancer. The tongue pressure measurement device currently used in our center is multipurpose; it is used for evaluation, reevaluation (e.g., posttreatment assessment), and lingual functional training exercises to gain tongue muscle strength. This device also provides positive feedback, increasing exercise motivation.

In summary, all of the above-described new instrumental swallowing tools have clinical capability in the diagnosis of oropharyngeal dysphagia. Information obtained from these new techniques augments the current intensive research and active rehabilitation strategies used in the clinical care of patients with dysphagia.

Appendix

Other Available Dysphagia Screening Tools

These time- and cost-effective tools are used to identify patients at high risk of dysphagia who therefore require further assessment. Two recent systematic reviews [8, 42] of dysphagia impairment identified the following two validated and reliable screening tools based on sufficient sample sizes and accepted psychometric criteria for clinical use in stroke survivors:

1. Toronto Bedside Swallowing Screening Test (TOR-BSST©)
2. Barnes Jewish Hospital Stroke Dysphagia Screen

TOR-BSST© [4, 43, 44]

The TOR-BSST© is a stable and accurate dysphagia screening tool for patients with stroke. It is one of the highest-ranking dysphagia screening tools and is quick and easy to perform, taking less than 10 min to administer and score [42]. The TOR-BSST© can be administered by any healthcare professional (e.g., nurse, dietician) who has received training by an SLHT using a standardized training program. The test consists of three sections: the first two sections involve an oral examination (tongue movement and voice quality), and the third section involves a series of water swallow tests. A patient who has failed any section of the test stops the screening and is referred to an SLHT for further evaluation.

The TOR-BSST© has demonstrated high validity; the sensitivity of the trial swallow using water and the negative predictive value were 96.35% and 93.30%, respectively, in the acute setting and 80.00% and 89.50%, respectively, in the rehabilitation setting. The inter-rater reliability for administration was excellent, with an intraclass correlation coefficient of 0.92 (95% confidence interval, 0.85–0.96). However, the TOR-BSST© is copyrighted and must be purchased before administration. Its purchase includes online training and information on how to implement the screening protocol, which may be desirable for some facilities.

Barnes Jewish Hospital Stroke Dysphagia Screen [45, 46]

The Barnes Jewish Hospital Stroke Dysphagia Screen is a simple 2-min bedside screening test for acute stroke patients. It involves measurement of the level of consciousness, assessment of several items that indicate the presence of dysarthria (asymmetry or weakness in the facial, lingual, and palatal regions), and performance of a 3-oz water swallow test. This test showed high sensitivity (95%) using VF for concurrent validity, a high negative predictive value (94%), and moderate specificity (68%).

Martino et al. [9] performed another systematic review of bedside screening tools with which to detect oropharyngeal dysphagia in patients with neurological disorders. The authors identified two clinical screening tools that met the methodological quality assessment requirements (validity, reliability, and generalizability) and had high sensitivity with moderate specificity:

1. Volume-Viscosity Swallowing Test
2. TOR-BSST©, described above

Volume-Viscosity Swallowing Test [47]

The Volume-Viscosity Swallowing Test was designed to identify clinical signs of impaired swallowing efficacy and safety. This test is also used to select the appropriate bolus volume and viscosity with which to achieve the highest safety and efficacy of deglutition by testing three viscosities (nectar, liquid, and pudding).

Many other screening methods administered in different settings are available for clinical use, including the 3-oz water swallow test described by Suiter and Leder [48], the Gugging Swallowing Screen described by Trapl et al. [49], the Burke Dysphagia Screening Test described by DePippo et al. [50], and others.

As in bedside screening, protocols may vary among bedside tests with different goals and among different clinical settings, number of trial swallows, chosen cutoff points for aspiration or penetration, or bolus consistencies and volumes tested. At present, no guideline or consensus exists with respect to the most effective protocol in any screening procedure.

References

1. Donovan NJ, Daniels SK, Edmiaston J, Weinhardt J, Summers D, Mitchell PH. Dysphagia screening: state of the art: invitational conference proceeding from the State-of-the-Art Nursing Symposium, International Stroke Conference 2012. Stroke. 2013;44(4):e24–31. doi:10.1161/STR.0b013e3182877f57.
2. Martino R, Foley N, Bhogal S, Diamant N, Speechley M, Teasell R. Dysphagia after stroke: incidence, diagnosis, and pulmonary complications. Stroke. 2005;36(12):2756–63.
3. Hinchey JA, Shephard T, Furie K, Smith D, Wang D, Tonn S. Formal dysphagia screening protocols prevent pneumonia. Stroke. 2005;36(9):1972–6.
4. Martino R, Pron G, Diamant N. Screening for oropharyngeal dysphagia in stroke: insufficient evidence for guidelines. Dysphagia. 2000;15(1):19–30.
5. Lakshminarayan K, Tsai AW, Tong X, Vazquez G, Peacock JM, George MG, et al. Utility of dysphagia screening results in predicting poststroke pneumonia. Stroke. 2010;41(12):2849–54. doi:10.1161/STROKEAHA.110.597039.
6. Daniels SK, Anderson JA, Willson PC. Valid items for screening dysphagia risk in patients with stroke: a systematic review. Stroke. 2012;43(3):892–7. doi:10.1161/STROKEAHA.111.640946.
7. Baba M, Saitoh E, Takeda S, Onogi K. Swallowing evaluation for accommodation of oral feeding. Sogo Rehabil. 2002;30:1309–16. (Japanese).
8. Kertscher B, Speyer R, Palmieri M, Plant C. Bedside screening to detect oropharyngeal dysphagia in patients with neurological disorders: an updated systematic review. Dysphagia. 2014;29(2):204–12. doi:10.1007/s00455-013-9490-9.
9. Martino R, Flowers HL, Shaw SM, Diamant NE. A systematic review of current clinical and instrumental swallowing assessment methods. Curr Phys Med Rehabil Rep. 2013;1:267–79. doi:10.1007/s40141-013-0033-y.
10. Poorjavad M, Jalaie S. Systemic review on highly qualified screening tests for swallowing disorders following stroke: validity and reliability issues. J Res Med Sci. 2014;19(8):776–85.
11. Oguchi K, Saitoh E, Mizuno M, Baba M, Okui M, Suzuki M. The repetitive saliva swallowing test (RSST) as a screening test of functional dysphagia (1) normal values of RSST. Jpn J Rehabil Med. 2000;37:375–82. (Japanese).
12. Oguchi K, Saitoh E, Baba M, Kusudo S, Tanaka T, Onogi K. The repetitive saliva swallowing test (RSST) as a screening test of functional dysphagia (2) Validity of RSST. Jpn J Rehabil Med. 2000;37:383–8. (Japanese).
13. Tohara H, Saitoh E, Mays KA, Kuhlemeier K, Palmer JB. Three tests for predicting aspiration without videofluorography. Dysphagia. 2003;18(2):126–34.
14. Saitoh E. Grant for Ministry of Welfare (Comprehensive Gerontologic Science) Comprehensive study of treatment and management for dysphagia. Report of Grant for Ministry of Welfare. 2009;1999:1–18.

15. Kubota T, Mishima H, Hanada M, Minami I, Kojima Y. Paralytic dysphagia in cerebrovascular disorder – screening tests and their clinical application. Sogo Rehabil. 1982;10:271–6. (Japanese).
16. Horiguchi S, Suzuki Y. Screening tests in evaluating swallowing function. Jpn Med Assoc J. 2011;54(1):31–4.
17. Takeda S, Saitoh E, Matsuo K, Baba M, Fujii W, Palmer JB. Influence of chewing on food transport and swallowing. Jpn J Rehabil Med. 2002;39(6):322–30.
18. Ozaki K, Kagaya H, Yokoyama M, Saitoh E, Okada S, González-Fernández M, et al. The risk of penetration or aspiration during videofluoroscopic examination of swallowing varies depending on food types. Tohoku J Exp Med. 2010;220(1):41–6.
19. The government revision of medical fee. The fourth version of VF standard procedure (detail version). Jpn J Dysphagia Rehabil. 2014;18(2):166–86. https://www.jsdr.or.jp/wp-content/uploads/file/doc/VF18-2-p166-186.pdf. (Japanese).
20. Rosenbek JC, Robbins JA, Roecker EB, Coyle JL, Wood JL. A penetration-aspiration scale. Dysphagia. 1996;11(2):93–8.
21. Wright RER, Boyd CS, Workman A. Radiation doses to patients during pharyngeal videofluoroscopy. Dysphagia. 1998;13:113–5.
22. Crawley MT, Savage P, Oakley F. Patient and operator dose during fluoroscopic examination of swallow mechanism. Br J Radiol. 2004;77:654–6.
23. Zammit-Maempel I, Chapple CL, Leslie P. Radiation dose in videofluoroscopic swallow studies. Dysphagia. 2007;22:13–5.
24. Kanamori D, Kagaya H, Fujii N, Inamoto Y, Nakayama E, Suzuki S, et al. Examination of the distance measurement error and exposed dose when using a 320-row area detector CT: a comparison with videofluoroscopic examination of swallowing. Jpn J Compr Rehabil Sci. 2011;2:18–23.
25. Langmore S. Endoscopic evaluation and treatment of swallowing disorders. 2nd ed. New York: Thieme; 2001.
26. Wu CH, Hsiao TY, Chen JC, Chang YC, Lee SY. Evaluation of swallowing safety with fiberoptic endoscope: comparison with videofluoroscopic technique. Laryngoscope. 1997;107(3):396–401.
27. Hiss SG, Postma GN. Fiberoptic endoscopic evaluation of swallowing. Laryngoscope. 2003;113(8):1386–93.
28. Aviv JE, Kaplan ST, Thompson JE, Spitzer J, Diamond B, Close LG. The safety of flexible endoscopic evaluation of swallowing with sensory testing: an analysis of 500 consecutive evaluations. Dysphagia. 2000;15:39–44.
29. Warnecke T, Teismann I, Oslenber S, Hamacher C, Ringelstein EB, Schabitz WR, et al. The safety of fiberoptic endoscopic evaluation of swallowing in acute stroke patients. Stroke. 2009;40(2):482–6. doi:10.1161/STROKEAHA.108.520775.
30. Toda F, Kagaya H, Baba M, Shibata S, Ozeki Y, Kanamori D, et al. Effect of swallowing rounds on the outcome of dysphagic patients. Jpn J Compr Rehabil Sci. 2015;6:50–5.
31. Sellars C, Bowie L, Bagg J, Sweeney MP, Miller H, Tilston J, et al. Risk factors for chest infection in acute stroke: a prospective cohort study. Stroke. 2007;38(8):2284–91.
32. Armstrong JR, Mosher BD. Aspiration pneumonia after stroke: intervention and prevention. Neurohospitalist. 2011;1(2):85–93. doi:10.1177/1941875210395775.
33. Almeida SR, Bahia MM, Lima FO, Paschoal IA, Cardoso TA, Li LM. Predictors of pneumonia in acute stroke in patients in an emergency unit. Arq Neuropsiquiatr. 2015;73(5):415–9. doi:10.1590/0004-282X20150046.
34. Fujii N, Inamoto Y, Saitoh E, Baba M, Okada S, Yoshioka S, et al. Evaluation of swallowing using 320-detector-row multislice CT. Part I: single- and multiphase volume scanning for three-dimensional morphological and kinematic analysis. Dysphagia. 2011;26(2):99–107. doi:10.1007/s00455-009-9268-2.
35. Inamoto Y, Fujii N, Saitoh E, Baba M, Okada S, Katada K, et al. Evaluation of swallowing using 320-detector-row multislice CT. Part II: kinematic analysis of laryngeal closure during normal swallowing. Dysphagia. 2011;26(3):209–17. doi:10.1007/s00455-010-9276-2.

36. Inamoto Y, Saitoh E, Okada S, Kagaya H, Shibata S, Ota K, et al. The effect of bolus viscosity on laryngeal closure in swallowing: kinematic analysis using 320-row area detector CT. Dysphagia. 2013;28(1):33–42.
37. Inamoto Y. Swallowing disorder - Kinematic analysis and understanding of dysphagia pathophysiology using swallowing CT. Innervation. 2014;29(5):73–6.
38. Inamoto Y, Saitoh E. Novel swallowing evaluation using swallowing CT. Jon J Rehabil Med. 2015;52:36–41.
39. Okada T, Aoyagi Y, Inamoto Y, Saitoh E, Kagaya H, Shibata S, et al. Dynamic change in hyoid muscle length associated with trajectory of hyoid bone during swallowing: analysis using 320-row area detector computed tomography. J Appl Physiol. 2013;115:1138–45. doi:10.1152/japplphysiol.00467.2013.
40. Shibata S, Kagaya H, Inamoto Y, Saitoh E, Okada S, Ota K, et al. Swallowing maneuver analysis using 320-row area detector computed tomography (320-ADCT). Jpn J Compr Rehabil Sci. 2011;2:54–62.
41. Nakayama E, Kagaya H, Saitoh E, Inamoto Y, Hashimoto S, Fujii N, et al. Changes in pyriform sinus morphology in the head rotated position as assessed by 320-row area detector CT. Dysphagia. 2013;28(2):199–204. doi:10.1007/s00455-012-9430-0.
42. Schepp SK, Tirschwell DL, Miller RM, Longstreth WT Jr. Swallowing screens after acute stroke: a systematic review. Stroke. 2012;43(3):869–71. doi:10.1161/STROKEAHA.111.638254.
43. Martino R, Silver F, Teasell R, Bayley M, Nicholson G, Streiner DL, et al. The Toronto Bedside Swallowing Screening Test (TOR-BSST): development and validation of a dysphagia screening tool for patients with stroke. Stroke. 2009;40(2):555–61. doi:10.1161/STROKEAHA.107.510370.
44. SCORE (Stroke Canada Optimization of Rehabilitation through Evidence) evidence-based recommendations for the upper and lower extremities and risk assessment post-stroke 2007. Ottawa: Canadian Stroke Network; 2007. http://www.canadianstrokenetwork.ca/eng/tools/downloads/SCORE_EBR_Aug2307.pdf. Accessed 19 Oct 2015.
45. Edmiaston J, Connor LT, Loehr L, Nassief A. Validation of a dysphagia screening tool in acute stroke patients. Am J Crit Care. 2010;19(4):357–64. doi:10.4037/ajcc2009961.
46. Edmiaston J, Connor LT, Ford AL. SWALLOW-3D, a simple 2-minute bedside screening test, detects dysphagia in acute stroke patients with high sensitivity when validated against videofluoroscopy (abstract). Stroke. 2011;42:e352.
47. Clavé P, Arreola V, Romea M, Medina L, Palomera E, Serra-Prat M. Accuracy of the volume-viscosity swallow test for clinical screening of oropharyngeal dysphagia and aspiration. Clin Nutr. 2008;27(6):806–15. doi:10.1016/j.clnu.2008.06.011.
48. Suiter DM, Leder SB. Clinical utility of the 3-ounce water swallow test. Dysphagia. 2008;23(3):244–50.
49. Trapl M, Enderle P, Nowotny M, Teuschl Y, Matz K, Dachenhausen A, et al. Dysphagia bedside screening for acute-stroke patients: the Gugging Swallowing Screen. Stroke. 2007;38(11):2948–52.
50. DePippo KL, Holas MA, Reding MJ. The Burke dysphagia screening test: validation of its use in patients with stroke. Arch Phys Med Rehabil. 1994;75(12):1284–6.

Part III
Treatment

Chapter 6
Oral Hygiene Care

Yoko Inamoto, Kannit Pongpipatpaiboon, Seiko Shibata, Yoichiro Aoyagi, Hitoshi Kagaya, and Koichiro Matsuo

Abstract People with dysphagia are at a greater risk of poor oral hygiene and health. Dried secretion accumulated in oral cavity reduces oral sensitivity and promote bacterial growth. Aspiration of these pathogens can lead to life-threatening respiratory disorders and pulmonary infection. Oral care is therefore important issue from the perspective of preventing aspiration pneumonia and swallowing rehabilitation in dysphagic patients.

A growing amount of scientific evidence is showing that oral health care is strongly correlated with aspiration pneumonia [1, 2]. Many reports have addressed the importance of regular oral care in preventing pneumonia by eliminating bacterial colonization in the oral cavity, preventing dental decay, and maximizing the ability to eat safely and comfortably [3–7]. This is true in both dysphagic patients and older people who cannot independently manage their oral care. Improving or maintaining proper swallowing and oral function is important from the perspective of retaining patients' quality of life [8].

Patients with oral dryness (xerostomia) due to reduced salivary flow (e.g., patients who cannot feed orally, have a lower level of consciousness, or are being treated with certain medications) are very high risk of developing complex oral diseases and dental problems. Xerostomia yields many negative consequences

Y. Inamoto (✉)
Faculty of Rehabilitation, School of Health Sciences, Fujita Health University, Toyoake, Aichi, Japan
e-mail: inamoto@fujita-hu.ac.jp

K. Pongpipatpaiboon • S. Shibata • Y. Aoyagi • H. Kagaya
Department of Rehabilitation Medicine I, School of Medicine, Fujita Health University, Toyoake, Aichi, Japan
e-mail: ning665@gmail.com; sshibata@fujita-hu.ac.jp; yyy@rc5.so-net.ne.jp; hkagaya2@fujita-hu.ac.jp

K. Matsuo
Department of Dentistry, School of Medicine, Fujita Health University, Toyoake, Aichi, Japan
e-mail: kmatsuo@fujita-hu.ac.jp

E. Saitoh et al. (eds.), *Dysphagia Evaluation and Treatment*,
https://doi.org/10.1007/978-981-10-5032-9_6

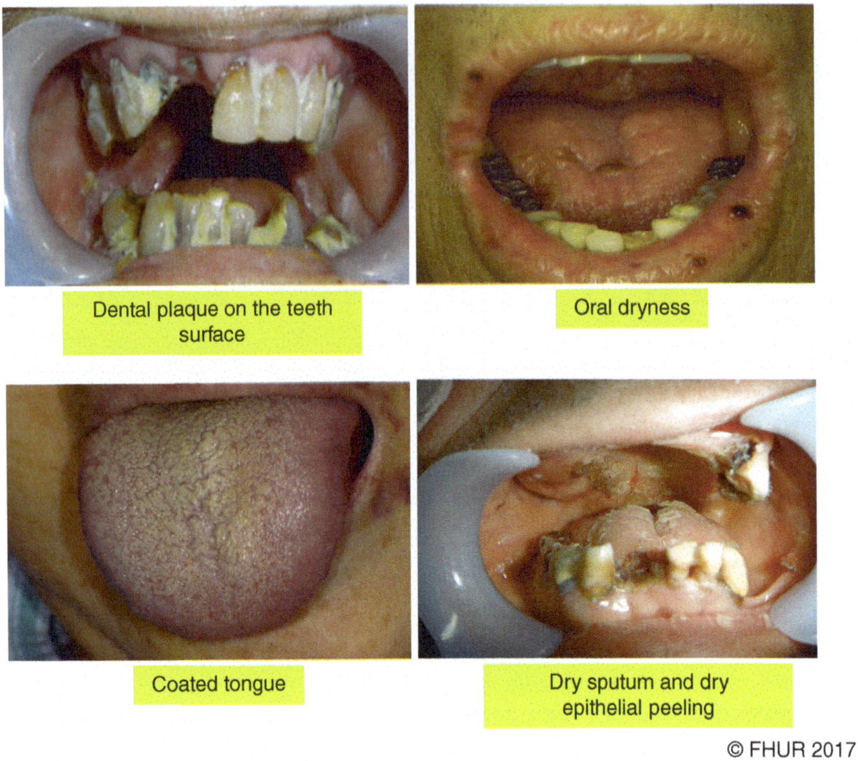

Fig. 6.1 Common oral problems in dysphagic patients and older people

including insufficient food bolus formation and transport, mucosal ulceration, demineralization of the dentition, dental caries, altered oral flora, and loss of appetite secondary to impaired taste and smell [9, 10]. Dry secretions that accumulate on the tongue and palate reduce oral sensitivity and promote bacterial growth, increasing the risk of upper respiratory infection and thus aspiration pneumonia [11, 12]. The concept of oral health care includes not only oral cleaning but also eating stimulation (Fig. 6.1).

Assessment of the patient's dental and oral hygiene status is necessary during the clinical examination, after instrumental investigation with boluses and swallowing rehabilitation training. If necessary, appropriate treatment such as dental treatment and oral hygiene care is carried out.

Missing teeth and poorly fitted dentures predispose the patient to aspiration because these conditions often exhibit chewing difficulty which consequently leads the poor coordination with the bolus formation, transportation, and swallowing. Infected teeth and poor oral hygiene predispose the patient to aspiration of contaminated oral secretions, leading to pneumonia. Although tube-fed patients do not feed orally, many studies have shown that feeding tubes do not prevent aspiration of contaminated oral secretions, refluxed enteral foods, or regurgitated gastric contents. One research group evaluated 19 observational cohort studies with respect to the correlation between the duration of feeding tube placement and the proportion of patients free of aspiration pneumonia and found that a nothing per os status provided no protection against aspiration pneumonia [13].

Therefore, to prevent aspiration pneumonia, clinicians must consider oral hygiene care and how to prevent aspiration in patients who do not feed orally. Additionally, patients with impairments of oral function such as those with hemiparalyzed oral structures (e.g., lips, tongue, soft palate) experience poor mastication, poor bolus formation, and accumulation of oral residue, all of which increase the risk of aspiration and poor swallowing outcomes.

At FHUR, dentists and dental hygienists play a major role in oral hygiene and dental care. The oral care protocol at FHUR was developed by dentists, dental hygienists, and certified nurses in dysphagia in cooperating with nursing staff in other disciplines, particularly the neurology unit, geriatric unit, pulmonary unit, and otolaryngology head and neck cancer unit (Fig. 6.2).

Additionally, the Japanese version of the Oral Health Assessment Tool is utilized for dental and oral health screening. This tool includes eight categories: lips, tongue, gums and tissues, saliva, natural teeth, dentures, oral cleanliness, and dental pain. The score for each category is divided into three levels: 0 = healthy, 1 = oral changes, and 2 = unhealthy. These scores are summed to obtain the total score, the maximum of which is 16 (Fig. 6.3).

The oral care screening is mostly performed by ward nurses. Patients with a high Oral Health Assessment Tool score, poor dentition, a poor oral status, or the need for further examination and intensive oral care are referred to the dental department. Dentists then individually examine, treat, and prescribe oral hygiene care that is carried out by a dental hygienist.

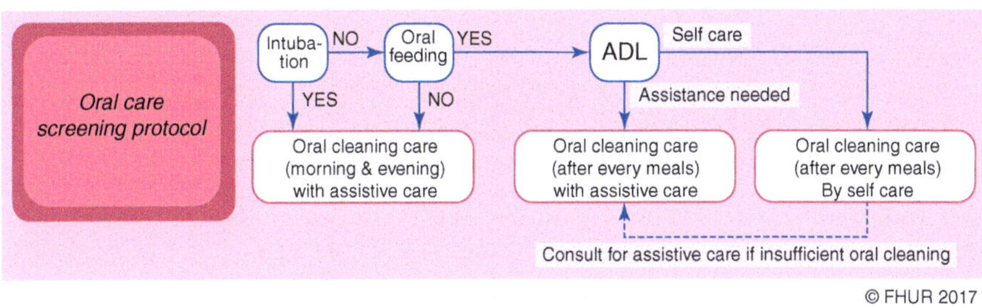

Fig. 6.2 Oral care protocol at Fujita Health University Rehabilitation Complex

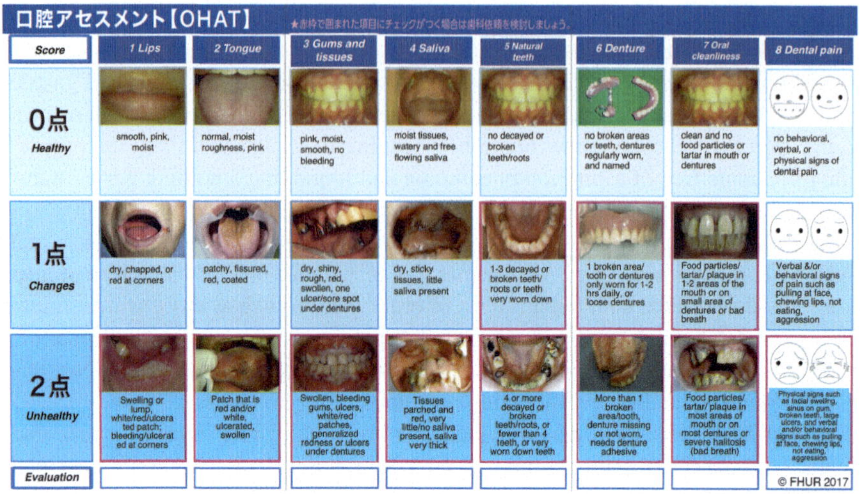

Fig. 6.3 Oral Health Assessment Tool (OHAT) for dental and oral health assessment screening

The oral care protocol involves mechanical cleaning and elimination of contaminants. This is achieved through the following steps (also shown in Fig. 6.4):

1. Oral moisturizing gel is first applied to the lips and then to the soft surfaces of the oral cavity to moisturize and soften any dried or hard secretions.
2. The teeth are manually brushed without a dentifrice; an interdental brush is used if necessary.
3. Softened contaminants are removed with a sponge brush.
4. The tongue is cleaned with a tongue scraper by scraping from the back to the front of the tongue surface.
5. The palate and other soft tissues are mechanically cleaned with a sponge swab.
6. The presence of residual contaminants in the oral cavity is rechecked; if present, they are eliminated by wiping to prevent their entrance into the pharynx (and thus decrease the risk of aspiration) and decrease the level of bacteria following oral care. Because dysphagic patients can easily aspirate rinsing water, wiping the oral cavity with mouth wipes (wet tissue wrapped around a finger) is recommended for all parts of the oral cavity including the teeth, gums, tongue, and palate.
7. A moisturizing gel is applied to the soft tissues of the oral cavity.

In summary, poor oral hygiene predisposes patients to aspiration of contaminated oral secretions, leading to pneumonia. Providing regular dental and oral hygiene care and cleaning can lower the risk of aspiration pneumonia. Therefore, the development of an oral care protocol and maintenance care system is a critical step to enhance eating function and prevent pneumonia in patients with dysphagia.

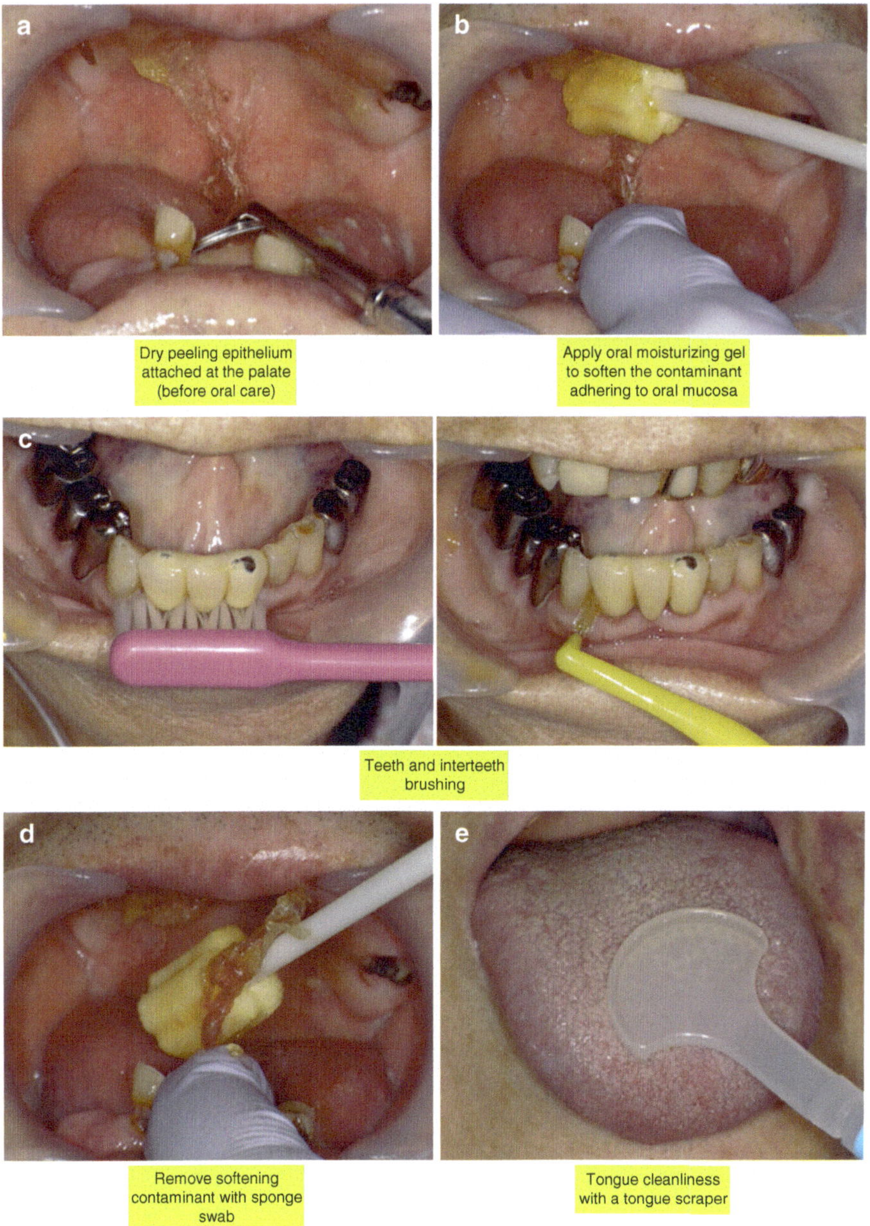

Fig. 6.4 Oral care protocol

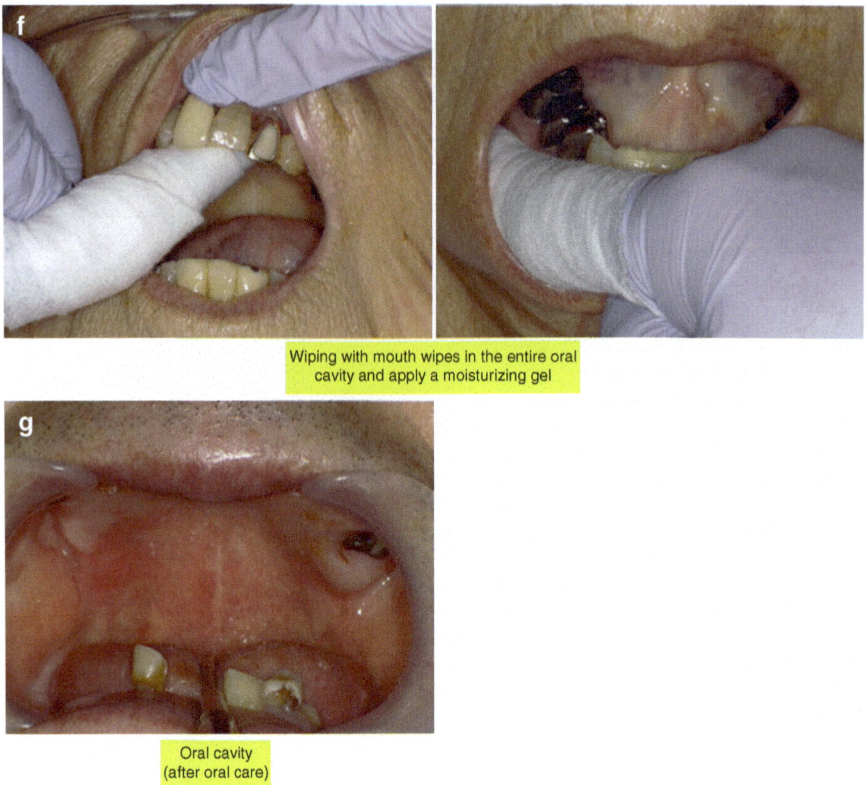

Fig. 6.4 (continued)

References

1. Terpenning M. Geriatric oral health and pneumonia risk. Clin Infect Dis. 2005;40(12):1807–10.
2. Fernández OO, Clavé P. Oral hygiene, aspiration, and aspiration pneumonia: from pathophysiology to therapeutic strategies. Curr Phys Med Rehabil Rep. 2013;1:292–5. doi:10.1007/s40141-013-0032-z.
3. Terpenning MS, Taylor GW, Lopatin DE, Kerr CK, Dominguez BL, Loesche WJ. Aspiration pneumonia: dental and oral risk factors in an older veteran population. J Am Geriatr Soc. 2001;49(5):557–63.
4. Yoneyama T, Yoshida M, Ohrui T, Mukaiyama H, Okamoto H, Hoshiba K, et al. Oral care reduces pneumonia in older patients in nursing homes. J Am Geriatr Soc. 2002;50(3):430–3.
5. Sørensen RT, Rasmussen RS, Overgaard K, Lerche A, Johansen AM, Lindhardt T. Dysphagia screening and intensified oral hygiene reduce pneumonia after stroke. J Neurosci Nurs. 2013;45(3):139–46. doi:10.1097/JNN.0b013e31828a412c.
6. Ikeda M, Miki T, Atsumi M, Inagaki A, Mizuguchi E, Meguro M, et al. Effective elimination of contaminants after oral care in elderly institutionalized individuals. Geriatr Nurs. 2014;35(4):295–9. doi:10.1016/j.gerinurse.2014.03.003.
7. Ortega O, Parra C, Zarcero S, Nart J, Sakwinska O, Clavé P. Oral health in older patients with oropharyngeal dysphagia. Age Ageing. 2014;43(1):132–7. doi:10.1093/ageing/aft164.

8. El-Solh AA. Association between pneumonia and oral care in nursing home residents. Lung. 2011;189(3):173–80. doi:10.1007/s00408-011-9297-0.
9. Zlotnik Y, Balash Y, Korczyn AD, Giladi N, Gurevich T. Disorders of the oral cavity in Parkinson's disease and parkinsonian syndromes. Parkinsons Dis. 2015;2015:379482. doi:10.1155/2015/379482.
10. Furuta M, Yamashita Y. Oral health and swallowing problems. Curr Phys Med Rehabil Rep. 2013;1(4):216–22.
11. Clavé P, Shaker R. Dysphagia: current reality and scope of the problem. Nat Rev Gastroenterol Hepatol. 2015;12(5):259–70. doi:10.1038/nrgastro.2015.49.
12. Wirth R, Dziewas R, Beck AM, Clavé P, Hamdy S, Heppner HJ, et al. Oropharyngeal dysphagia in older persons – from pathophysiology to adequate intervention: a review and summary of an international expert meeting. Clin Interv Aging. 2016;11:189–208. doi:10.2147/CIA.S97481.
13. Finucane TE, Bynum JP. Use of tube feeding to prevent aspiration pneumonia. Lancet. 1996;348(9039):1421–4.

Chapter 7
Swallowing Exercises

Yoko Inamoto, Kannit Pongpipatpaiboon, Seiko Shibata, Yoichiro Aoyagai, Hitoshi Kagaya, and Koichiro Matsuo

Abstract Before describing the swallowing exercises in this chapter, we first address the principle of such exercises. This fundamental knowledge provides a comprehensive understanding of the term "exercise" and the techniques by which to achieve effective treatment outcomes. The swallowing exercise-based treatment will be described based upon the principle of rehabilitation medicine for which its target aims to achieve functional improvement through the changes of physiological impairment.

The main goal of rehabilitation medicine is reconstruction of life. This is achieved by systematic integration of four methodologies: comprehensive medical management, the activity-function-structure relationship, therapeutic learning, and the assistive system (Fig. 7.1).

The activity-function-structure relationship refers to the fact that function and structure are adjusted based on the activity level. Basically, immobilization or disuse syndrome leads to deterioration of many body functions and the development of various diseases. In contrast, encouragement of activity with early rehabilitative intervention helps to prevent disuse syndrome and gain functional ability by the overload principle. A greater load than normally experienced on the body can enhance the ability of activity-dependent elements (e.g., muscle strength, range of motion) that are used for daily activities and contribute to functional improvement (Fig. 7.2).

Y. Inamoto (✉)
Faculty of Rehabilitation, School of Health Sciences, Fujita Health University, Toyoake, Aichi, Japan
e-mail: inamoto@fujita-hu.ac.jp

K. Pongpipatpaiboon • S. Shibata • Y. Aoyagai • H. Kagaya
Department of Rehabilitation Medicine I, School of Medicine, Fujita Health University, Toyoake, Aichi, Japan
e-mail: ning665@gmail.com; sshibata@fujita-hu.ac.jp; yyy@rc5.so-net.ne.jp; hkagaya2@fujita-hu.ac.jp

K. Matsuo
Department of Dentistry, School of Medicine, Fujita Health University, Toyoake, Aichi, Japan
e-mail: kmatsuo@fujita-hu.ac.jp

E. Saitoh et al. (eds.), *Dysphagia Evaluation and Treatment*,
https://doi.org/10.1007/978-981-10-5032-9_7

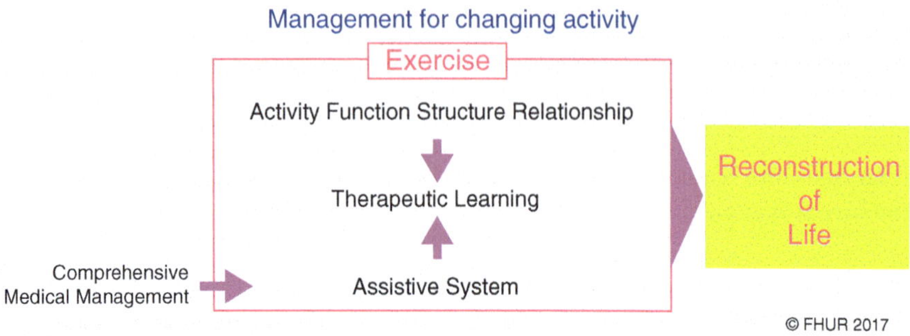

Fig. 7.1 Four main methodologies that comprise the core components of rehabilitation exercise: comprehensive medical management, the activity-function-structure relationship, therapeutic learning, and the assistive system

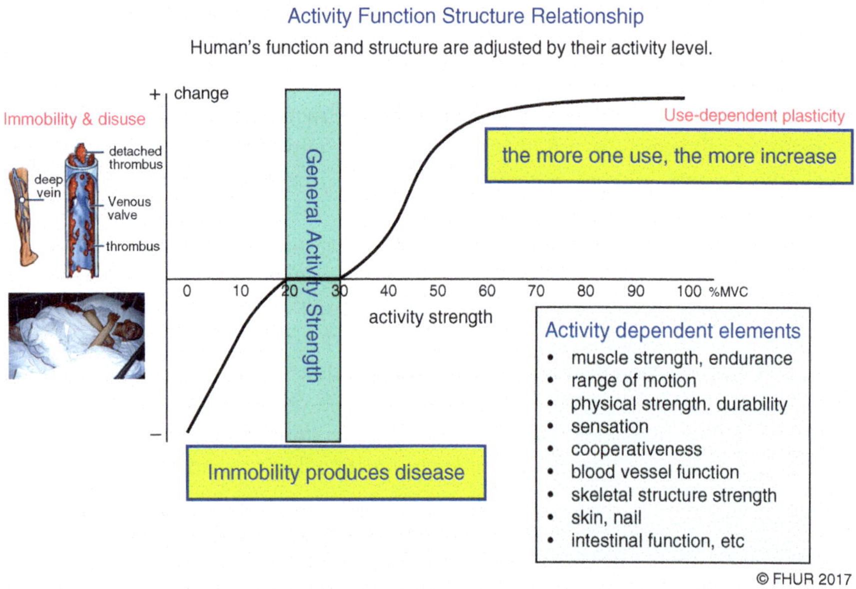

Fig. 7.2 Activity-function-structure relationship

The assistive system comprises instrumental aspects (e.g., modified dysphagia food, swallowing chair, dental prosthesis) and environmental aspects (e.g., social resources, family support, environment). To achieve the reconstruction of life in rehabilitation medicine, instruments and the environment are utilized effectively. Therapeutic learning is the motor learning process in which target behavior is achieved by utilizing activity-dependent elements and the assistive system.

7.1 Successful Rehabilitation Strategies Based on Motor Learning in Patients with Swallowing Disorders

Motor learning refers to how motor performance is improved and subsequently maintained. Motor learning is defined as a set of processes that are associated with practice or experience and that lead to relatively permanent changes in the capability for skilled performance [1]. The principle of motor learning is based on a limb movement system emphasizing kinematic assessment through feedback during training. It integrates activity-dependent factors and environment to learn new activities using critical tasks.

7.1.1 Evaluation of Rehabilitation Strategies Based on Motor Learning

A motor learning curve is a graphical representation of the increases of learning skill (vertical axis) with exercise (horizontal axis). The plot shows a patient's motor improvement while performing a task repeatedly. A large number of individual trials during training eventually increase the task proficiency and result in a skillful experience to recovery of the patient's functional capacity (Fig. 7.3).

A motor learning curve, especially with respect to skill proficiency, displays three phases of performance changes associated with task difficulty:

Too difficult: If a task is too difficult (or the ability of the patient is too low to perform the task), the rehabilitation progress is very slow. The performance training

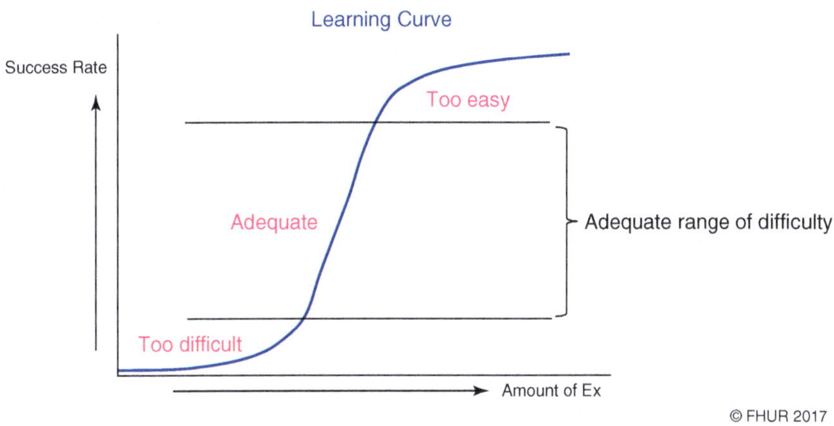

Fig. 7.3 Motor learning curve indicating the patient's ability and exercise dose

may fail, and the patient is unable to become proficient. Consequently, the patient may experience loss of motivation and lethargy during the training program.

Adequate: The ability of the patient to approach the optimal level of task performance is helpful for rapid progression in training. The possibility of success in this phase is around 70%. A proper task difficulty level allows the patient to further improve his or her motor skill.

Too easy: Once a patient practices a too-easy task for which he or she has already reached a certain level of motor skill, the progress plateaus within the learning curve.

The most effective way to achieve successful performance in motor learning must be considered. The principle of motor learning comprises four key factors.

1. Transferability (task specificity)

Transferability refers to the probability that the patient can transfer from performance of a training task to achievement of the final targeted area or function. Similarity between the training task and target task is important.

2. Motivation (psychological driving force)

Motivation should be considered situation-dependent, and the patient should receive reinforcement from either intrinsic or extrinsic resources.

3. Performance change (behavioral modification)

There are three major components to acquiring relatively permanent motor skills:

a. Feedback

Feedback is composed of knowledge of results and knowledge of performance; both influence the motor learning process:

- *Knowledge of results* is feedback regarding the results, indicating limit-difficulty tasks and the success of activity with respect to overall performances (e.g., the result of VF study showing penetration, aspiration, or pharyngeal residue).
- *Knowledge of performance* is feedback that provides specific information regarding the performance strategy, such as food modifications, postural modification, and the effect of swallowing maneuvers. This feedback can reinforce exercise training or the application of the swallow maneuver for dysphagia treatment.

b. Quantity (amount/frequency of exercise)

High numbers of repetitions (repetitive tasks) are essential to the success of motor learning. The number of repetitions performed in a given exercise protocol is based on the progression and regimen used in training. Repetition is a very important key for improvement. According to the overload principle, when the threshold of the target intensity is reached, the patient will gain both activity-dependent elements and skill acquisition.

c. Difficulty of exercise

Difficulty should be kept in mind when choosing the appropriate task to ensure that an exercise is effective, as mentioned in the description of the skill proficiency curve. The task that fits the patient's level (not too easy and not too difficult) can be transferable to the target.

Three essential components to overcome task difficulty are:

- Task selection (proper bolus consistency and volume depending on the patient's pathophysiological disorders)
- Instrumental usage (e.g., assistive devices)
- Rehabilitation techniques (e.g., facilitation techniques, swallowing maneuvers)

These components will be further clarified in the discussion of treatment.

4. Retention/application

Exercise helps to maintain task performance. Additionally, high variability in task training and the performance of random tasks can improve retention.

7.2 Swallowing Exercises

After completion of treatment-oriented evaluations such as VE and VF, all information must be integrated and analyzed to determine the most appropriate treatment approach based on the individual patient's pathophysiological considerations. Notably, swallowing treatment is not "one-size-fits-all" therapy. Recognizing patients' individual pathophysiology allows for effective clinical decision-making in terms of what type of physiology-based exercise (intervention) is the most suitable. The principle of "different physiological disorders, different treatment interventions" is vital to dysphagia management.

When planning dysphagia treatment, clinicians must consider multiple factors:

- The definitive or most likely diagnosis
- The patient's general health status (stable/unstable, medical condition, cognitive condition)
- The patient's current swallowing ability and associated problems
- The patient's current nutritional status (type, amount, time)
- Previous and most recent evaluation and treatment
- Caregiver and social support

Table 7.1 Swallowing exercise-based rehabilitation therapies

Element-based exercise (activity-function-structure relationship)	Behavior-based exercise (therapeutic learning)
Oral element-based exercise • Lingual range-of-motion exercise • Lingual strengthening exercise • Lingual oromotor control exercise	*Facilitation technique (including similar effects)* • Thermal-tactile stimulation • K-point stimulation • Balloon dilatation
Pharyngeal elemental-based exercise • Shaker exercise • Tongue base exercise • Tongue-holding exercise (Masako maneuver)	*Target-oriented exercise* • Swallowing maneuvers 1. Supraglottic swallow 2. Super-supraglottic swallow 3. Mendelsohn maneuver 4. Effortful swallow • Postural techniques (single, combine): trunk, head/neck • Diet modifications
Other Expiratory muscle-strengthening exercise	

This information is helpful for both planning therapeutic interventions and determining the proper time for initiation of swallowing rehabilitation on an individual-patient basis.

Swallowing exercises aim to achieve permanent functional improvement in swallowing through alterations of physiological impairment. In Japan, swallowing treatment is generally classified as indirect and direct exercises. Indirect exercise focuses on exercises performed without food or liquid as a part of the treatment program. In contrast, direct exercise is performed with utilization of food and/or liquid. This classification is introduced from the view of swallowing related to risk.

The Fujita swallowing team classifies the swallowing exercise based on the previously described principle of the four components of rehabilitation medicine as a reconstruction of activity (Fig. 7.1):

1. Element-based exercises (activity-function-structure relationship)
2. Behavior-based exercises (therapeutic learning)

The goal of element-based exercises is to increase the functional level of activity-dependent elements such as muscle strength and endurance, range of motion, and coordination of structures. The goal of behavior-based exercises is to integrate activity-dependent elements with swallowing activity through the learning. In this type of exercise, swallowing behavior is more strongly emphasized and performed with a suitable level of difficulty (Table 7.1).

Decisions regarding therapeutic strategies should be based on accurate evaluation and diagnosis of swallowing disorders, ideally identifying physiological impairments by VF and/or VE study. The following section of text presents the details of each exercise used for dysphagic patients at FHUR.

7.2.1 *Element-Based Exercises*

Element-based exercises target neuromotor control, which is a prerequisite for swallowing function. Knowledge of the activity-function-structure relationship is fundamental for a comprehensive understanding of the effects of swallowing interventions. The particular structure that corresponds to the targeted function must be considered. An understanding of this relationship will help clinicians to easily determine the most appropriate treatment plan for the patient (Fig. 7.4).

7.2.1.1 Oral Element-Based Exercises

- Organs: lower jaw, lip, cheek, and tongue
- Functions: bolus intake, mastication, bolus formation, and bolus propulsion
- Training: range-of-motion exercise, strengthening exercises (resistant and endurance), and oromotor control exercises

The tongue is the key component in oral element-based exercises and plays the most important role in oropharyngeal swallowing, especially in the oral stage, which involves oral preparatory functions and oral transit. The major roles of the tongue are bolus intake, bolus holding, mastication, bolus formation, and bolus propulsion. Thus, tongue exercises are essential for improvements in the swallowing functional outcome. Many types of exercises are used to improve tongue function and are described below.

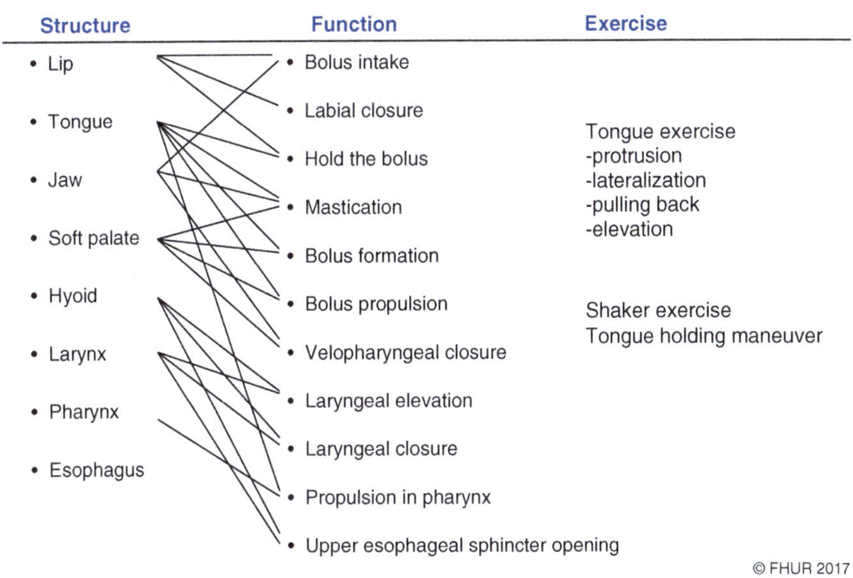

Fig. 7.4 Relationship between structure and function as the basis of element-based exercises

Tongue range-of-motion exercises are fundamental for bolus manipulation in both the oral preparation and transit stages. All directions of tongue movement are important, including elevation from the front to the back, lateralization, protrusion, and pulling back. During tongue movement in each direction, the clinician asks the patient to hold the tongue in a particular position for a few seconds. A gradual increase in frequency and intensity is necessary for functional improvement (Appendix "Tongue Range-of-Motion Exercise"). These exercises also promote tongue strengthening for bolus formation and propulsion, particularly the tongue blade elevation exercise. In addition to manual exercises, several devices are used to facilitate tongue strength (Appendices "Tongue Resistance-Strengthening Exercise" and "Devices to Facilitate Tongue Strengthening Exercise").

Oromotor control exercises are also important for oromotor function. These exercises involve not only the tongue but also other oral structures to promote improved bolus control (Appendix "Oromotor Control Exercise"). The clinician should gradually increase the speed of these exercises when the patient's ability has improved.

7.2.1.2 Pharyngeal Element-Based Exercises

- Organs: tongue base, hyoid bone, pharynx, larynx, and UES
- Functions: hyolaryngeal elevation, laryngeal closure, pharyngeal constriction, and UES dilatation
- Training: Shaker exercise, tongue base retraction exercise, and tongue-holding exercise (Masako maneuver)

Shaker Exercise

The Shaker exercise or head lift exercise is a combination of an isometric and isokinetic non-swallowing exercise to strengthen the suprahyoid muscles (specifically the geniohyoid, mylohyoid, and digastric muscles) and enhance thyrohyoid shortening. The physiologic principle of the Shaker exercise is an increase in superoanterior hyolaryngeal movement by strengthening of the suprahyoid muscles with a resultant improvement in UES opening [2]. One study revealed that the Shaker exercise was effective in patients who required tube feedings because of abnormal UES opening. The data showed a change in swallowing physiology with clinical improvement (reductions in pyriform sinus residue and post-swallowing aspiration) [3]. The Shaker exercise is recommended three times a day for 6 weeks; this results in a significant increase in the UES anteroposterior opening diameter and a decrease in the hypopharyngeal intrabolus pressure, which is a marker of flow resistance [4] (Appendix "Shaker Exercise"). This exercise protocol should be incrementally adjusted based on the patient's ability level. In some dysphagic patients with limited ability to perform the Shaker exercise (such as those with tracheostomy, severe weakness of head and neck muscles, limitation of neck movement, and/or inability to lift the head), strengthening of the suprahyoid muscles can be facilitated by alternative therapeutic interventions such as the jaw-opening exercise [5] (Appendix "Jaw-Opening Exercise").

Tongue Base Retraction Exercise

Tongue base retraction generates pressure with which to drive the pharyngeal bolus. The tongue base drives bolus material through the pharynx by moving back, making complete contact with the pharyngeal wall and thus applying pharyngeal pressure to the tail of the bolus. Therefore, tongue base retraction plays a critical role in pharyngeal clearance especially in the vallecula, acting in cooperation with pharyngeal constriction. The tongue base retraction exercise is designed to improve the maximum range of posterior movement of the tongue base, establishing strength to propel the bolus and ensure clearance of the bolus through the pharynx (Appendix "Tongue Base Retraction Exercise").

For patients who cannot follow the instructions provided by the clinician, the patient can pull the tongue back against the pulling force provided by the clinician at the tip of the tongue. Alternative therapies include voluntary tongue base strengthening exercises to improve impaired tongue base movement (e.g., gargling, yawning) [6].

Tongue-Hold Swallow Exercise (Masako Maneuver)

Contraction of the posterior pharyngeal wall coupled with posterior movement of the tongue base during swallowing provides the driving force necessary to assist bolus clearance, propelling the bolus through the upper pharynx during swallowing. Upper pharyngeal or vallecular residue is observed when insufficient contact is present between the tongue base and posterior pharyngeal wall.

The tongue-hold swallow exercise focuses specifically on pharyngeal contraction by physiologically increasing the anterior movement of the pharyngeal musculature (the superior pharyngeal constrictor muscle, the muscle fibers of which are in conjunction with the intrinsic muscles of the tongue), thus contributing to improved contact between the tongue base and posterior pharyngeal wall during the pharyngeal stage of swallowing [7–9] (Appendix "Tongue-Holding Swallow Exercise (Masako Maneuver)"). This exercise, therefore, is thought to aim for strengthening the pharyngeal contraction.

Because of the negative consequences of the tongue-hold maneuver, this exercise should not be performed with a bolus or during meals; it should instead be performed with saliva. Increased pharyngeal residue, a shortened duration of airway closure, and a longer pharyngeal swallow response time have been reported with the use of a bolus in dysphagic patients [10].

7.2.1.3 Other Exercises

Expiratory Muscle-Strengthening Exercise

The expiratory muscles function in respiration, speech, and voice production. Likewise, they have a potential role in swallowing function by enhancing the ability to perform a productive cough as a defense mechanism. This prevents material from entering the airway by providing adequate expiratory or subglottic pressure.

The expiratory muscle-strengthening exercise (EMST) is a non-swallowing exercise designed to modify the physiological biomechanisms of expiratory tasks related to swallowing function for airway protection in dysphagic patients. The therapeutic goal of the EMST is to improve the maximal expiratory pressure, cough strength, and subglottic pressure, all of which are associated with the coordination of swallowing function and help to reduce the risk of penetration and aspiration [11, 12]. Therefore, the EMST could translate to functional improvement in coughing and swallowing. At FHUR, we use two types of handheld airway clearance devices: the Portex Acapella® (Smiths Medical Inc., Minato-ku, Tokyo) and the Threshold positive expiratory pressure device (CHEST M.I., Inc., Bunkyo-ku, Tokyo). These devices combine the resistive feature of a positive expiratory pressure device with the vibratory feature of a flutter valve to mobilize retained airway secretions. Clearing the airway before swallowing training promotes safe swallowing and minimizes the risk of aspiration (Appendix "Expiratory Muscle Strengthening Exercise").

7.2.2 *Behavior-Based Exercises*

Behavior-based exercises promote therapeutic learning by integrating all the activity-dependent elements to the actual swallowing behavior by utilizing assistive system. The key of behavior-based exercises involves the task difficulty range. The difficulty of a task is one of the main components in motor learning that influences the possibility of achieving the targeted result. Methods with which to overcome difficult tasks include:

1. *Providing an easier task* that can be transferable to the target (e.g., postural techniques, food modifications, swallowing maneuvers)
2. *Changing conditions* (e.g., facilitative techniques)

The proper method will provide an adequate range of task difficulty and promote achievement of the desired goal (Fig. 7.5).

The combination of both facilitation techniques and target-oriented exercises ensures the most effective swallowing treatment. For example, postural strategies, diet modification, and/or swallowing maneuvers are manipulated to contribute to the difficulty of a task; this is performed along with stimulation technique during the swallowing exercises, as shown in Fig. 7.6. Once a patient's condition has improved, the task should be modified toward a higher goal based on the patient's success rate.

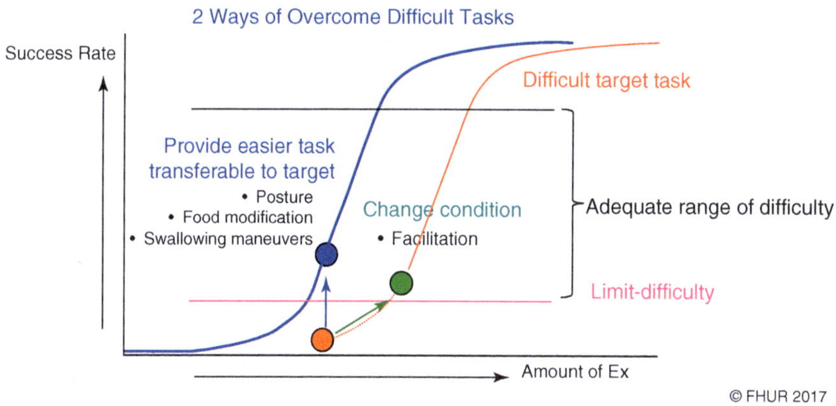

Fig. 7.5 Two methods to overcome difficult tasks based on behavioral exercise

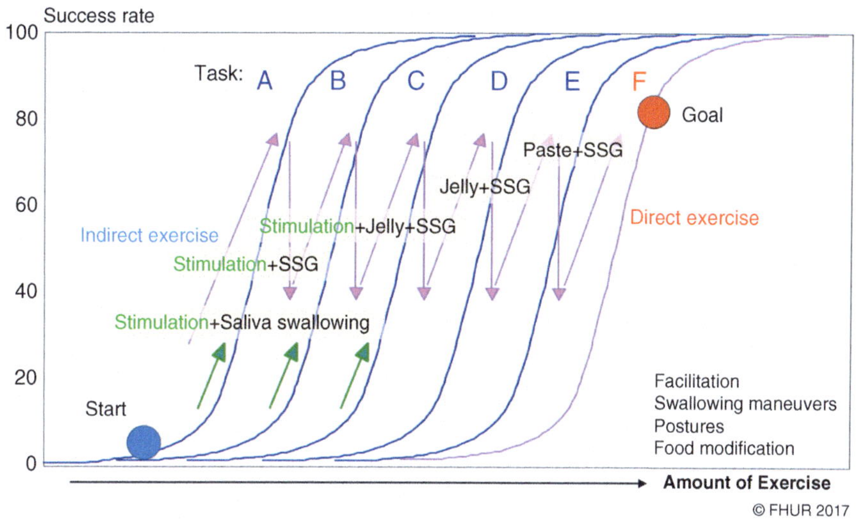

Fig. 7.6 Exercise task with consideration of task difficulty

7.2.2.1 Facilitation Techniques (Including Similar Effects)

Facilitation induces a temporary change in the patient's ability and encourages successful performance of the swallowing exercise. The three most common facilitation techniques are thermal-tactile stimulation, K-point stimulation, and the balloon dilatation exercise.

Thermal-Tactile Stimulation [3, 6, 13]

Thermal-tactile stimulation is a sensory stimulation technique most commonly used to improve triggering of the pharyngeal swallow in patients with a delayed swallowing reflex and high risk of pre-swallow airway invasion resulting from this delay.

The purpose of cold mechanical stimulation is to heighten the oral sensitivity for the swallow and possibly alter central nervous system excitability by stimulus-induced cortical plasticity. Cold application also acts as a sensory stimulus to the brain stem, inducing improvements in the swallowing physiology, which requires the ability to voluntarily swallow without stimulation.

The anterior faucial pillars are particularly recommended for mechanical thermal stimulation because they are one of the most sensitive oral areas for triggering of the swallowing reflex (Appendix "Thermal-Tactile Stimulation"). Thermal-tactile stimulation is performed on both sides in case of bilaterally equal sensitivity. Other areas in the oral cavity are also used to stimulate initiation of the swallow response during training, including the tongue base, posterior part of the tongue, velum, and posterior pharyngeal wall.

K-Point Stimulation [14]

K-point stimulation is a swallowing facilitation technique developed by Kojima in 2002. The K-point is located on the mucosa lateral to the palatoglossal arch and medial to the pterygomandibular fold at the height of the post-retromolar pad (Fig. 7.7).

This trigger point can be stimulated by a soft touch or light pressure applied by the clinician's finger or a tongue depressor to facilitate swallowing. K-point stimulation mechanically induces a pathological reflex, particularly in patients with pseudobulbar or suprabulbar palsy. The effects of pathological trigger point stimulation at the K-point in patients with pseudobulbar palsy include facilitation of the swallowing reflex with mastication-like movement and easier opening of the mouth in patients with trismus. Although K-point stimulation has a temporary effect, it allows patients to efficiently relearn actual swallowing exercises.

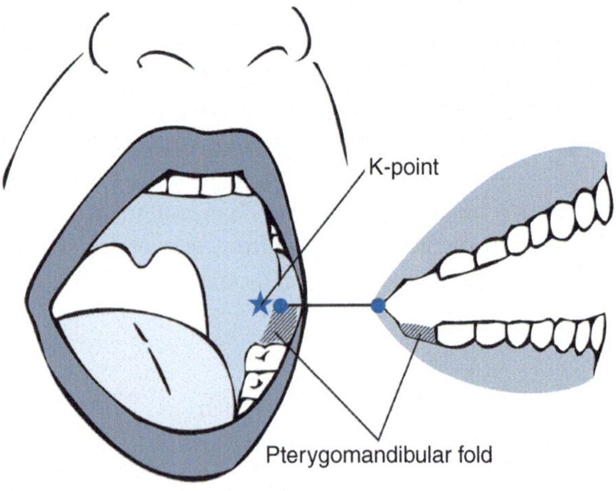

Fig. 7.7 The K-point is located on the mucosa lateral to the palatoglossal arch and medial to the pterygomandibular fold at the height of the post-retromolar pad (Reproduced from [42] with permission)

In Japan, a special device called the K-Spoon (Aoyoshi Co., Ltd., Niigata, Japan) is often used for K-point stimulation (Appendix "K-Spoon"). The K-point can be gently stimulated either before or during feeding by placing food from the K-Spoon onto the dorsum of the tongue and then touching the K-point with the tip of the K-Spoon, particularly in patients with a delayed swallowing reflex. The K-point can also be touched during bolus formation if oral movement has stopped while chewing.

Balloon Dilatation

Balloon dilatation, first reported in 1997 [15], is an optional conservative treatment widely used for cricopharyngeal dysfunction, particularly in patients with a large amount of post-swallowing pharyngeal residue in the pyriform sinus [15–17]. This procedure is cost-effective, minimally invasive, safe, and generally well-tolerated. This balloon-expanding procedure works by stretching the cricopharyngeal muscle and surrounding tissues, facilitating the relearned coordinated swallowing process between UES relaxation and pharyngeal contraction, and improving the sensory-motor coordination of the UES [16, 17]. The balloon dilatation technique is demonstrated in Appendix "Balloon Dilatation" (Figs. 7.8 and 7.9).

At FHUR, balloon dilatation is first performed under VF to ensure accurate positioning of the dilated balloon at the UES, determine the immediate effect of balloon dilatation, and obtain biofeedback of the performance. A round balloon is used (Foley, 12–14 Fr). VF is performed twice, before and immediately after balloon dilatation, to evaluate bolus flow through the UES. After confirmation of the tolerability and immediate effects, balloon dilatation is performed at the bedside by SLHTs. The initial volume of air blown into the balloon is 3–4 ml; this is gradually increased to 10 ml based on the patient's condition. Balloon dilatation is usually performed 5–10 times per set (2–3 sets/day).

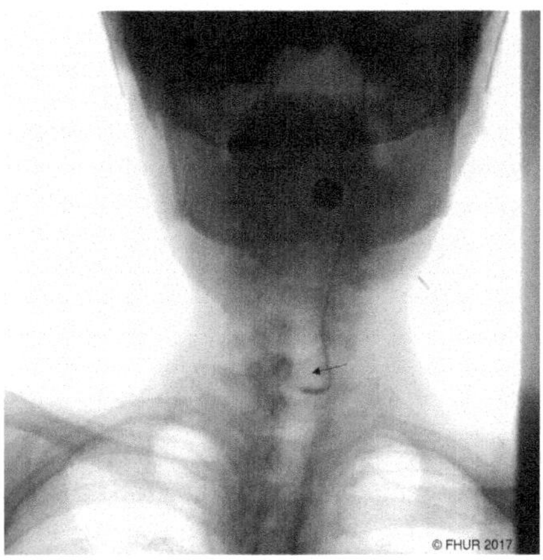

Fig. 7.8 Pulling of the balloon (*arrow*) backward through the UES during VF (*anteroposterior view*)

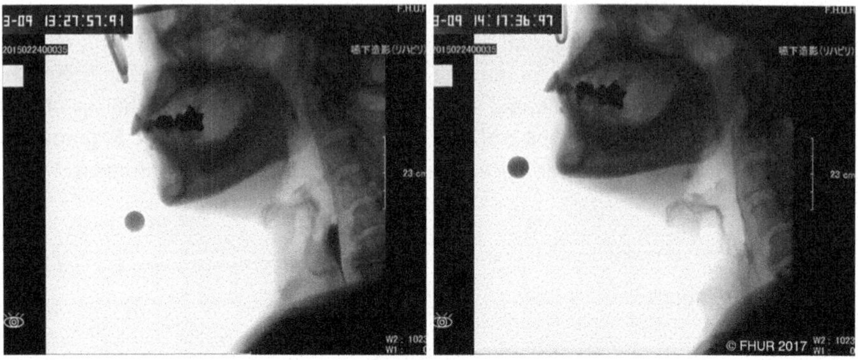

Fig. 7.9 Lateral fluoroscopic view, (*left*) before balloon dilatation; bolus residue is present in the pyriform sinus after swallowing, (*right*) after balloon dilatation; no bolus residue is present after swallowing

7.2.2.2 Target-Oriented Exercises

Target-oriented exercises involve repeated performance of easier, limit-difficulty tasks. Patients can become proficient after repeated practice. There are three aspects to overcoming task difficulty: swallowing maneuvers, postural strategies, and diet modifications.

Swallowing Maneuvers

Swallowing maneuvers involve the application of voluntary controls to a specific movement of the pharyngeal muscles used during swallowing [6]. These maneuvers change the swallow physiology, providing the patient with a new swallowing strategy. Several swallowing maneuvers are available, including the supraglottic and super-supraglottic swallow, Mendelsohn maneuver, and effortful swallow. Most maneuvers are difficult for patients to understand at their first attempt; thus, patients must persist with these exercises to become proficient. Swallowing maneuvers are generally initiated with a dry swallow followed by an actual bolus swallow; they are also used during meals to ensure swallow safety and efficacy. The recommended exercise protocol is usually at least 5–10 times per set, 2–3 sets per day, and 7 days per week. Additionally, VE or VF study can be used for visual performance feedback to enhance learning and examine the efficacy of the maneuvers.

Supraglottic and Super-Supraglottic Swallow

The supraglottic swallow and super-supraglottic swallow are volitional safe swallowing techniques used before and during the swallow for patients who demonstrate reduced airway protection secondary to delayed and/or decreased laryngeal closure.

Basically, laryngeal closure during swallowing involves approximation of valves including the true vocal folds, false vocal folds, and aryepiglottic folds as well as epiglottic inversion [18, 19]. Breath holding in both maneuvers facilitates earlier laryngeal closure and improves safe bolus passage. Breath holding prior to and throughout the swallow increases closure of the true vocal folds and medial approximation of the arytenoids, but the super-supraglottic swallow involves extra effort [18–21]. The extra effort involved in breath holding (super-supraglottic swallow) provides more effective and supplemental function for greater airway protection via closure of the false vocal folds and anterior tilting of the arytenoids toward the base of the epiglottis. Subsequent coughing after the swallow and before breathing again aims to clear any residual material that has entered the laryngeal vestibule during the swallow or material that has been aspirated upon opening of the vocal folds and inhalation (Appendix "Supraglottic and Super-Supraglottic Swallow").

Mendelsohn Maneuver

The Mendelsohn maneuver is designed to augment superior and anterior movement of the hyolaryngeal complex and the subsequent increase in the UES opening (both the anteroposterior opening diameter and opening duration) during swallowing [22, 23]. This maneuver also has the potential to improve the timing and coordination of swallowing in the pharyngeal stage with the improvement in pharyngeal clearance [24, 25]. Furthermore, this maneuver can generally be performed to strengthen and enhance hyolaryngeal movement. Clinically, the Mendelsohn maneuver may be difficult for patients to understand and accomplish. The clinician typically shows the patient how to execute the maneuver by palpating the laryngeal elevation during the swallow to augment understanding and detecting the distance and duration of laryngeal movement (Appendix "Mendelsohn Maneuver").

Effortful Swallow

The effortful swallow was developed to improve the posterior movement of the tongue base [26–29] and increase the degree of pharyngeal constriction during the swallow [30]. It is used for patients in an attempt to improve bolus clearance from the vallecula [6]. Physiologically, the ultimate goal is to increase propagation of the pharyngeal pressure secondary to facilitating bolus flow through the pharynx and UES (Appendix "Effortful Swallow").

Postural Modification

Postural modification involves behavioral interventions to adjust the difficulty of swallowing tasks. Two essential principles of postural management are changes in gravity (e.g., reclining) and space manipulation (e.g., head rotation, head/neck flexion) of the bolus path, which thus controls bolus flow (direction and speed) through the pharynx (Fig. 7.10).

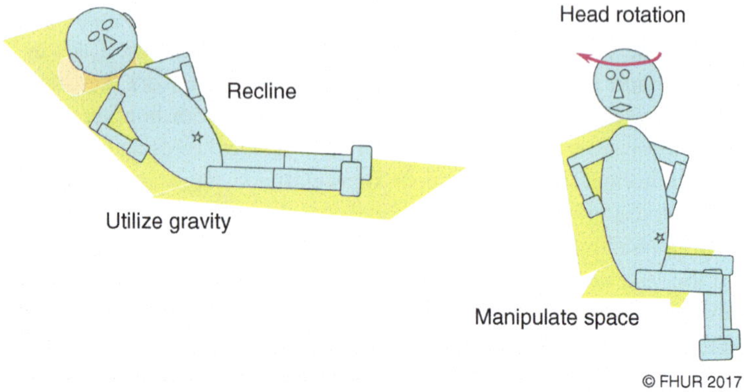

Fig. 7.10 Two key principles of postural management

Several postural strategies have been developed to minimize or eliminate the risk of food/liquid aspiration, enhance the efficiency of swallowing function, and maintain safe oral intake. Postural modification is often used in target-oriented exercise to augment swallowing function and is the first technique applied to prevent penetration or aspiration. This enables maintenance of a normal or near-normal diet and accelerates earlier removal of the feeding tube. It is easily utilized in combination with bolus modification to reduce the risk of aspiration. Before prescription of the postural adjustments, instrumental examination (especially VF) should be performed to precisely determine the efficacy of the postural strategies and the most appropriate texture and consistency of foods and fluids; this will allow the clinician to assess whether these strategies effectively reduce the risk of aspiration. The most common postural techniques used at FHUR, both during instrumental examination and swallowing training, are described below.

Reclining Position [31, 32]

The reclining or lying-down position is implemented to ensure a lower risk of aspiration than that associated with the seated-upright position. The reclining position changes the impact of gravity, affecting the bolus pathway and speed of bolus transport.

In the reclining position, with respect to the inclination of the oral cavity, the front of oral cavity is raised, and the back part is lowered. Thus, the bolus is transported easier from oral to the pharynx with the increased effect of gravity in oral cavity. Regarding the inclination of the posterior pharyngeal wall, the slope is getting moderate. Thus, the bolus advances slowly and arrives late at the hypopharynx with the decreased effect of gravity in the pharynx. Moreover, the trachea is positioned above the esophagus, resulting in a decreased incidence of the bolus entering the trachea and increasing the ability to hold the bolus in the pharynx without aspiration. Pharyngeal residue is likely to be held in the pyriform sinus, allowing patients to safely proceed with a second and third swallow and reducing the possibility of post-swallowing aspiration. This postural technique can be used in patients with impaired bolus transportation from the oral to the pharynx (e.g., bilateral reduction in pharyngeal wall contraction). The reclining technique is also useful in patients who have slow pharyngeal response.

The angle of the reclining position can be adjusted based on the patient's condition. A 30° reclining posture is often used for patients with severe dysphagia; this angle is then incrementally adjusted to ≥60°, which helps the patient to eat without any further assistance. Additionally, the impact of gravity in oral cavity must be considered. When the patient reclines, the speed of bolus flow in the oral cavity is accelerated. Severe oral phase problems such as poor bolus holding function may lead to premature spillage. Additionally, the head and neck position must be monitored while the patient is reclined to reduce the risk of aspiration secondary to an extended head and neck position. A pillow is thus recommended to maintain a flexed position.

Head Rotation or Head Turn

Head rotation is a postural strategy used to manipulate the hypopharyngeal space for control of the pharyngeal bolus flow through the esophageal inlet. Rotation of the head causes narrowing of the hypopharyngeal space on the rotated side and widening on the opposite, thus improving bolus clearance, i.e., a greater bolus volume is able to pass through the wider side of the bolus pathway [33, 34]. Accordingly, this postural compensatory technique is used for patients with pharyngeal hemiparesis, unilateral laryngeal dysfunction or reduced laryngeal closure, and impaired UES opening. Patients are instructed to turn their head to the weakened side as if they are looking over their shoulder (Fig. 7.11).

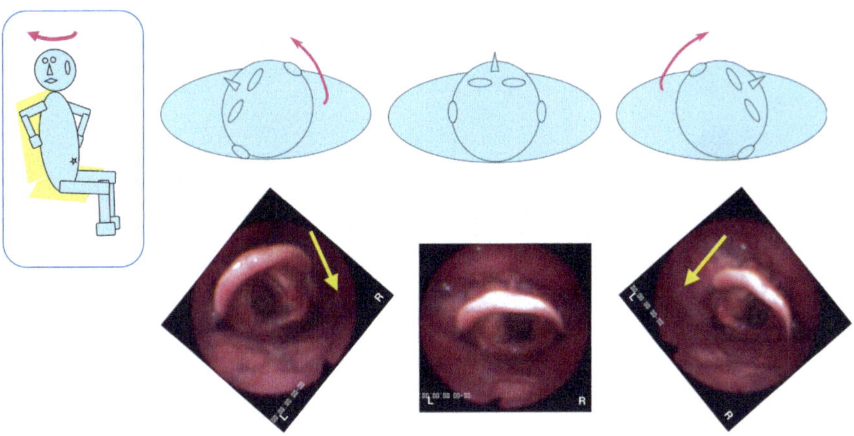

Fig. 7.11 VE images with a drawing of the head posture. Head rotation is performed to manipulate the hypopharyngeal space. The bolus proceeds along the wide passage on the opposite side of the rotated head (*arrow* in VE images)

Combination of Reclining and Head Rotation

When both gravity changes and space manipulation are needed to be utilized, reclining and head rotation are selected. However, caution is warranted. The bolus is transported to the rotated side of the head in the combined reclining and head rotation position because of the gravity effect. Thus, to prevent the bolus propulsion toward the rotated side of the head, trunk rotation to the opposite side of head rotation is necessary. For example, if the patient benefits from both right head rotation and reclining, left-side trunk rotation is required in combination with right head rotation and reclining (Figs. 7.12 and 7.13).

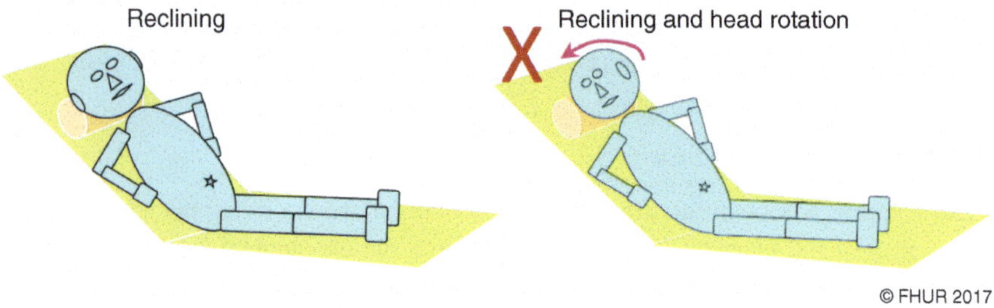

Fig. 7.12 *(Left)* reclining posture manipulates the bolus flow by the effect of gravity. *(Right)* the combination of reclining and head rotation in the semi-supine position may increase the risk of aspiration because of bolus going to the unintended right side due to the effect of gravity

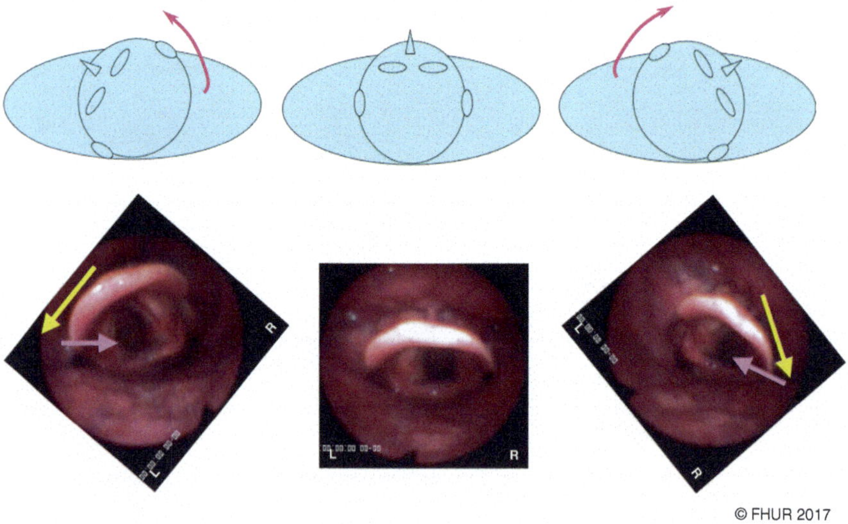

Fig. 7.13 VE images and a drawing of the combined posture (reclining and head rotation to the affected side). The bolus proceeds directly to the narrower side (head-rotated side) in accordance with the force of gravity, which may increase the risk of airway aspiration

Thus, to utilize both gravity and space manipulation for the purpose of reducing aspiration and residue, the postural approach involving combination of trunk rotation (side-lying) toward the sound side with head rotation to the paretic side along with reclining was developed. Rotating the body toward the unaffected side allows efficient downward movement of a bolus through the strong side with the help of gravity, and rotating the head toward the affected side widens the hypopharyngeal space on the unaffected side (Fig. 7.14).

Even if the effects of posture management are beneficial, actual performance of such manipulations may be difficult because of the need for multiple items, the inconsistent accuracy of the recommended posture, and patient fatigue or discomfort. These difficulties limit the postural effects and the swallowing ability of the patient. The swallowing chair was developed by Tomei Brace Co., Ltd. to overcome these barriers. This chair provides simplicity, ease, and comfort throughout the evaluation [35]. The swallowing chair also contributes to high reproducibility of postural adjustment within a short time. It can be easily adjusted with respect to both trunk reclining and rotating functions. Several accessories (including a pillow to support the head and neck, triangle pillows, a backrest, and leg guards) are available to achieve an accurate, stable, and comfortable posture to facilitate the patient's swallowing ability (Figs. 7.15 and 7.16).

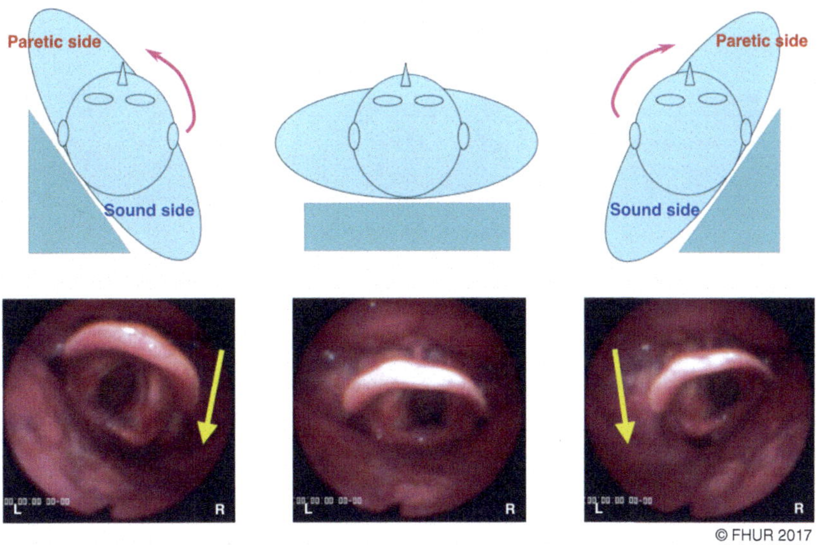

Fig. 7.14 VE images and a drawing of a combined posture: reclining, head rotation to the affected side, and trunk rotation to the unaffected side. The bolus advances to the sound side of the pharynx with the help of gravity, lessening the occurrence of airway aspiration

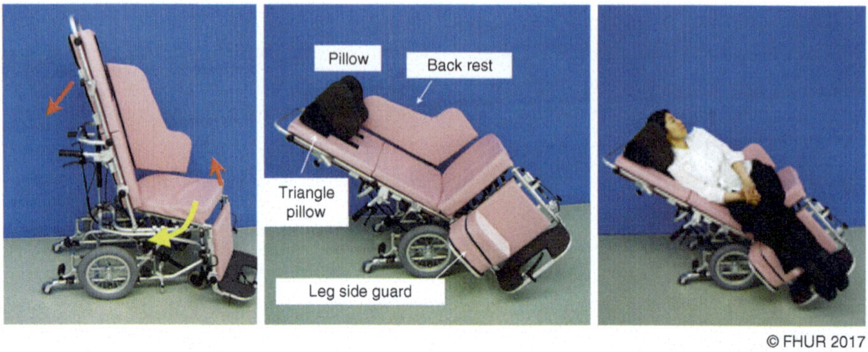

Fig. 7.15 The novel swallow chair. *(Left)* the swallow chair can be adjusted using reclining and tilting functions (*red arrow*) in addition to rotation of the seat by 30°, 60°, and 90° (*yellow arrow*). *(Middle)* accessories of the swallow chair provide rapid, accurate, and stable adjustment of posture; these include a pillow to hold the head and neck securely, triangle pillows, a backrest to provide back and hip stability, and leg guards to support the lower extremities. *(Right)* 30° reclining combined with right trunk rotation and left head rotation

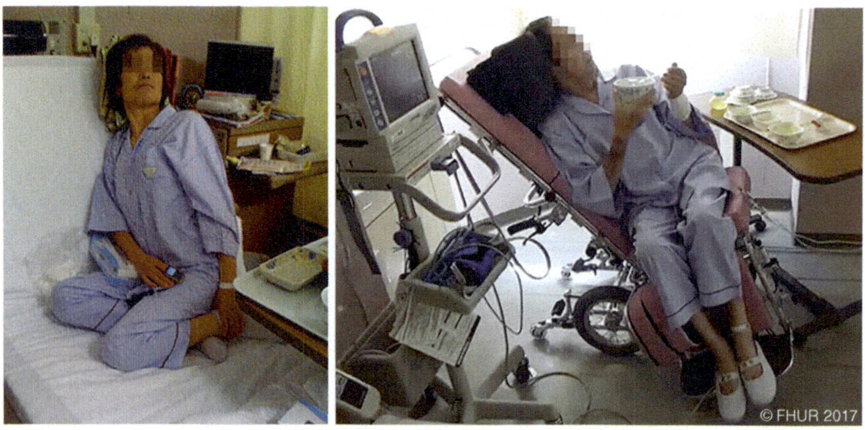

Fig. 7.16 Postural adjustment using the swallow chair (*right*) compared with the typical method on a bed (*left*), which seems uneasy and inconvenient. The use of the swallow chair promotes a more comfortable posture and facilitates the performance of swallowing exercises with safe oral intake

Head and Neck Flexion

Head and neck flexion is a postural technique used to adjust the pharyngeal space and is widely applied in dysphagia management. This maneuver has different physiological effects on different anatomical structures [36].

In head flexion, the whole upper cervical spine (occiput–C1, C1–C2) is flexed, pushing the tongue base and epiglottis backward and resulting in greater

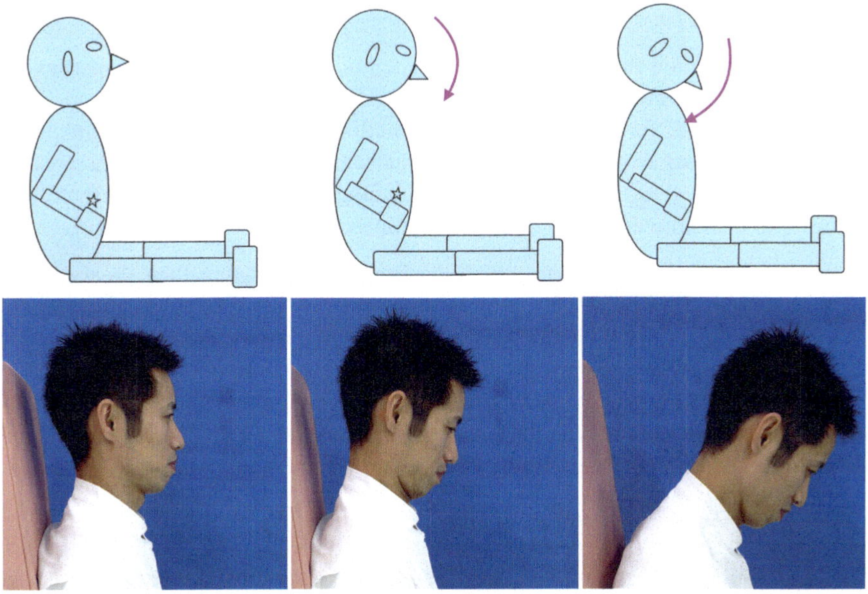

Fig. 7.17 Comparison of anatomical changes induced by head and neck flexion; (*left*) neutral position; (*middle*) head flexion, the neck is kept straight and the chin is tucked in and slightly downward; (*right*) neck flexion, the chin is brought toward the chest so that the patient is looking down at his or her knees

approximation of the tongue base with the posterior pharyngeal wall. This effect is useful for patients with bolus residue in the vallecula, which may cause post-swallowing aspiration. Conversely, in neck flexion, the middle and lower cervical spines (C2–C7) are flexed. Neck flexion widens the vallecula, which helps patients with a delayed swallowing reflex and prevents pre-swallowing aspiration. Combination of head and neck flexion is commonly performed to achieve safe oral feeding (Fig. 7.17).

Diet Modification (Texture Modification and Thickened Liquids)

Diet modification involves alteration of the consistency of foods and liquids to limit the difficulty of tasks, addressing both the safety and efficiency of swallowing. Modification of both the texture of foods and thickness of liquids has become a routine practice for the evaluation and treatment of swallowing difficulties. The next section of text clarifies the diet modification protocol performed at FHUR.

Texture-Modified Food

Texture modification involves mechanical alterations to the physical properties of food, changing the consistency (physical characteristics) of the original food. This diminishes the need for chewing or bolus formation, allows for easier consumption, and reduces the risk of serious health consequences such as choking and asphyxiation. The main food texture characteristics affecting bolus consistency and therefore the level of difficulty of swallowing are as follows:

1. *Cohesiveness*: The degree to which the food deforms rather than shears when compressed. This parameter reflects the ability of the food to form a united whole and withstand compression.
2. *Adhesiveness*: The effort necessary to overcome the attractive force of food that pulls it toward another contact surface (e.g., tongue, palate, teeth).
3. *Hardness (chewability)*: The force necessary to compress a food to attain a certain degree of deformation (e.g., biting and chewing a solid food just prior to shearing).

During the process of mastication and bolus formation, various physical properties (including chopping, mincing, grinding, and blending) of normally textured food are modified to achieve the safest food for the patient by softening, gathering the contents into one bite, and controlling the stickiness (Fig. 7.18).

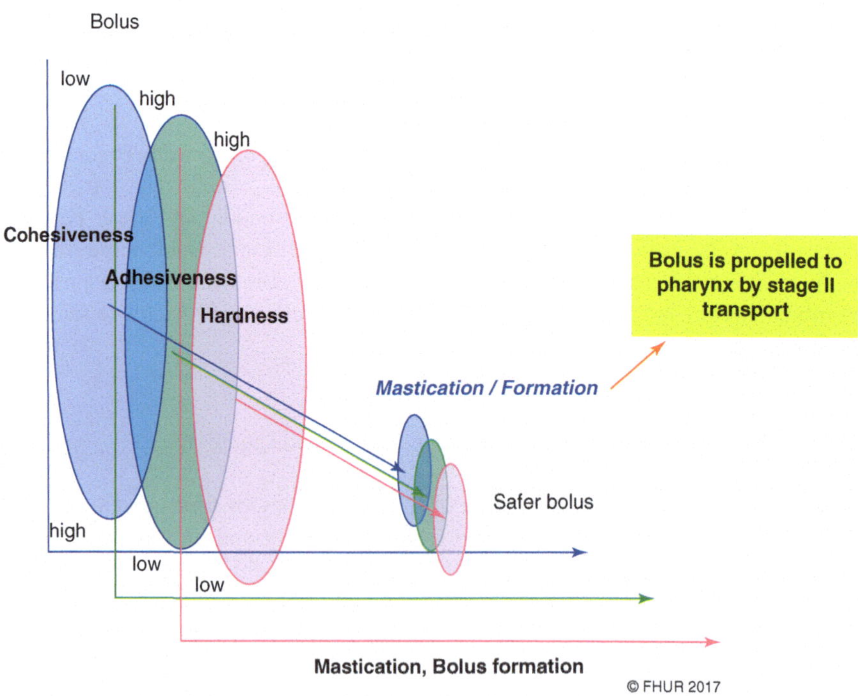

Fig. 7.18 Three main factors affecting bolus consistency (cohesiveness, adhesiveness, and hardness)

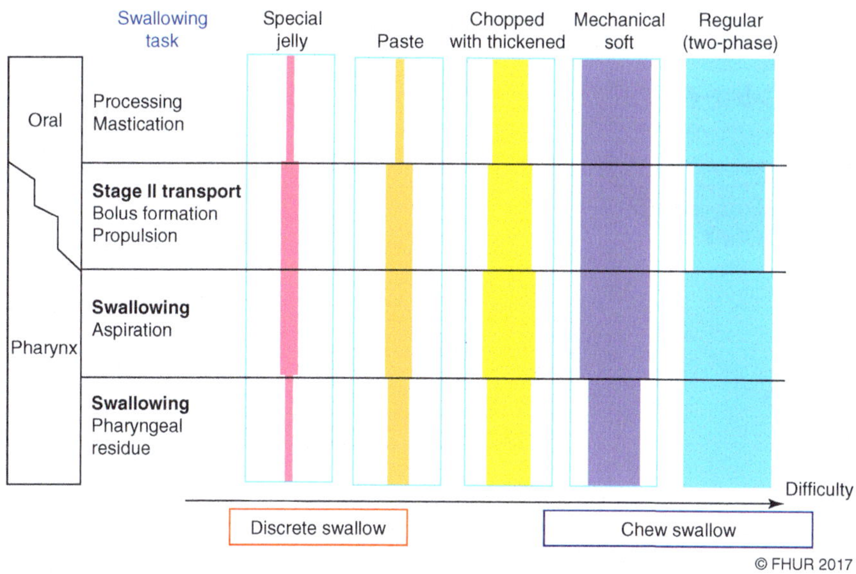

Fig. 7.19 Food difficulty adjustment of swallowing task in oral and pharyngeal stages. The width of the bar represents the difficulty level of the swallowing task

Based on the above concepts, the easiest and safest food to ingest is that requiring no chewing or change in bolus consistency. The bolus should be soft (low hardness), have good collectivity in the oral cavity and pharynx (high cohesiveness), and be able to be propelled without adhering to the mucous membrane (low adhesiveness), which is represented by special jelly (Engelead; Otsuka Pharmaceutical Factory, Inc.) [37].

Figure 7.19 shows the level of difficulty of food that has been modified for dysphagic patients with regard to the discrete and chew swallow. Both special jelly and paste have a homogeneous consistency that can be easily swallowed without chewing (discrete swallow), as shown by the very thin bar of the processing and mastication stages. Additionally, high cohesiveness and low adhesiveness help the safe transport with less likely to cause residue and aspiration. Notably, the special jelly does not melt into a liquid even when placed in the oral cavity and/or in the pharynx in a certain time of period. Thus, it is often used in the period of initial direct training as safest food (Fig. 7.20).

After paste, a chopped, thickened food is introduced; this requires a certain chewing ability (chew swallow) and increases the burden in the pharynx, resulting more risk of aspiration and residue. It is a potentially big step for patients with low swallowing ability, who comes to be able to manage paste food somehow. Ideally for the next step of paste food, food requiring certain ability of chewing and bolus formation in addition to have the same level of pharyngeal function for paste food is recommended. Because no actual food meets this description, the Fujita swallowing team collaborated with a company that developed a novel semisolid training

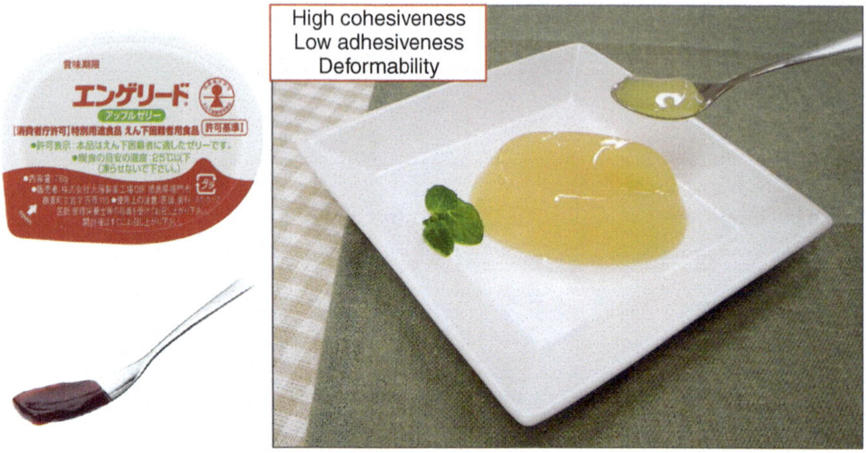

Fig. 7.20 Special jelly (Engelead) used in the initial period of direct swallowing training (Reproduced from Otsuka Pharmaceutical Factory, Inc. with permission)

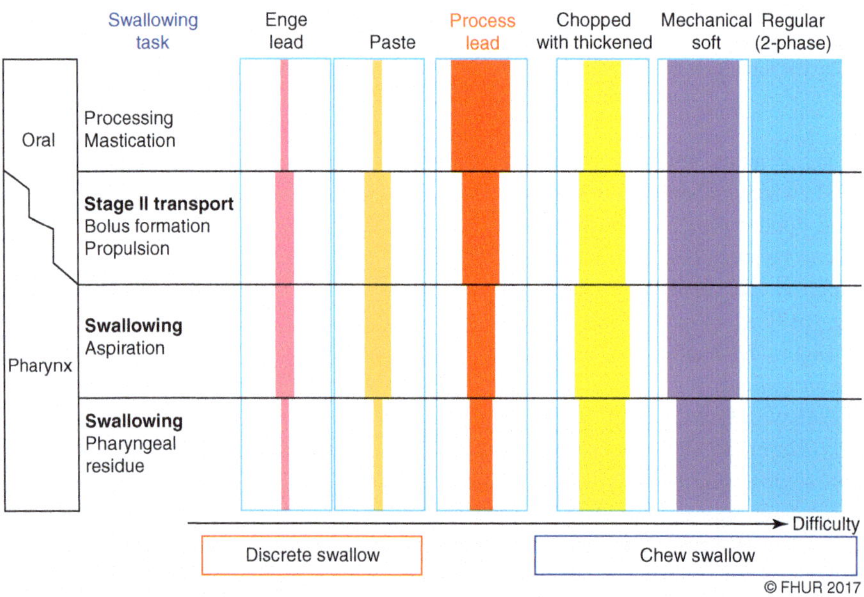

Fig. 7.21 Food difficulty adjustment for swallowing task. The process lead is available to practice processing and mastication in the oral stage with similar demand regarding bolus propulsion and swallowing ability in the pharyngeal stage

food, namely, a chew-swallow managing food (Process Lead; Otsuka Pharmaceutical Factory, Inc.) [38], as a training material based on the principle of mastication in the oral stage to provide the most appropriate food with respect to the swallowing task difficulty (Figs. 7.21 and 7.22).

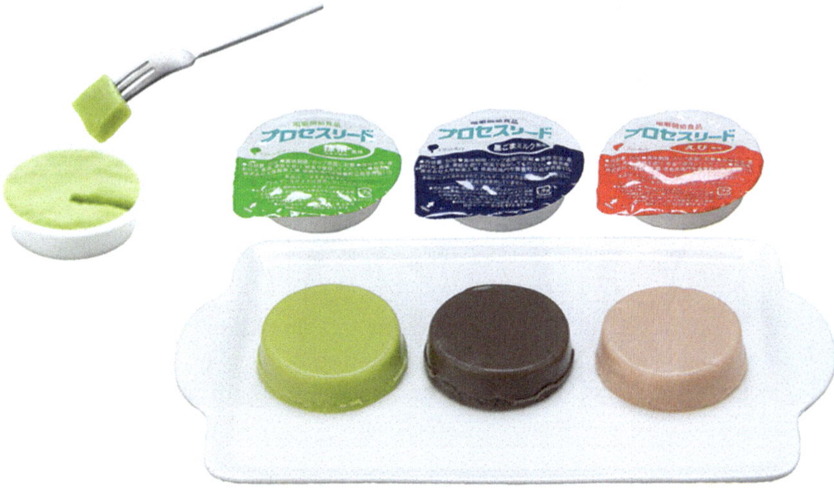

Fig. 7.22 Chew-swallow managing food/process lead for facilitation of the chew-swallow exercise. Although this food has an initial consistency and hardness requiring chewing, it is deformable, is easily coherent with saliva, can be readily propelled to the pharynx without adherence, and easily forms a bolus in the pharynx and collected in the vallecula with a texture equivalent to puree at the time of swallowing (Reproduced from Otsuka Pharmaceutical Factory, Inc. with permission)

At FHUR, we classify dysphagic food into six levels:

1. *Jelly diet*

   Uniform consistency (high cohesiveness and low adhesiveness) that can be swallowed as a single bolus
   Requires no chewing

2. *Paste diet*

   Homogeneous, high cohesiveness, and more variability of adhesiveness
   Requires no chewing

3. *Modified thickened diet*

   Consists of rice gruel and chopped softened food with thickened soup.
   A thickener is incorporated into all food in the meal.
   Bolus formation and transportation easily occur.
   Requires very little chewing.

4. *Mechanical soft diet*

   Consists of rice gruel and mechanical softened foods
   The mechanical softened food at a consistency that can be crushed by the gums or between the tongue and hard palate
   Requires some chewing

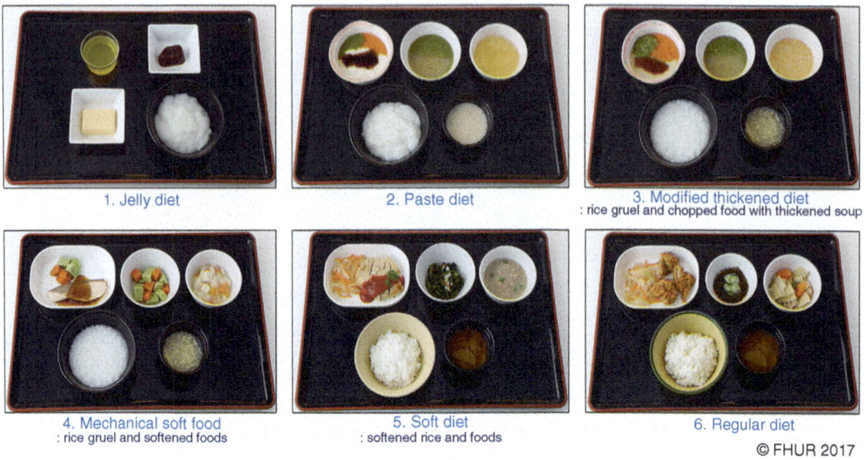
1. Jelly diet
2. Paste diet
3. Modified thickened diet
: rice gruel and chopped food with thickened soup
4. Mechanical soft food
: rice gruel and softened foods
5. Soft diet
: softened rice and foods
6. Regular diet
© FHUR 2017

Fig. 7.23 Six diet modification levels for dysphagic patients at Fujita Health University Hospital

5. *Soft diet*

   Consists of softened rice and foods

   The softened food at a consistency that requires a higher chewing ability than the mechanical softened food

6. *Regular diet (normal diet)*

   (Levels 4–6; liquid can be thickened with a thickener as necessary) (Fig. 7.23).

This classification system has been used to formulate diets of appropriate texture for individual dysphagic patients in our hospital and meets specific standards of swallowing safety. This food system is also used for direct swallowing training by SLHTs and nurses. Dieticians help to control the quality and consistency of dysphagia diets by ensuring adequate nutrient and energy contents.

New Innovation of Dysphagia Diet: Advanced Commercially Food Texture Modification in Japan

Advanced modification of commercial food has been developed with respect to various designs and tastes. This has been achieved by the enzyme homogeneous permeation technique, which produces precisely textured foods in terms of hardness and adhesiveness while maintaining the usual appearance of the original food [39] (Figs. 7.24 and 7.25).

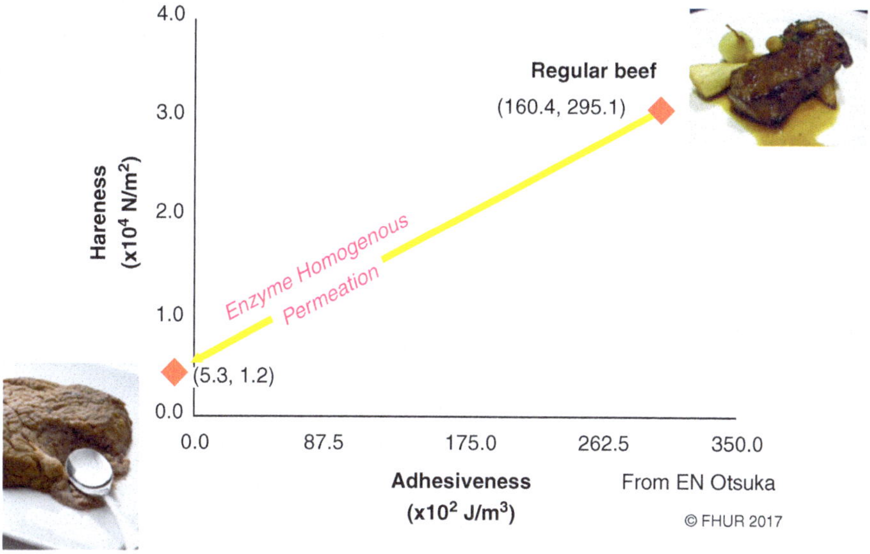

Fig. 7.24 Modified food in the form of a "beef steak" using the enzyme homogeneous permeation technique. Hardness has been converted from 160.4 to 5.3 × 10^4 N/m^2, and adhesiveness has been converted from 295.1 to 1.2 × 10^2 J/m^3 (EN Otsuka, Hanamaki, Japan)

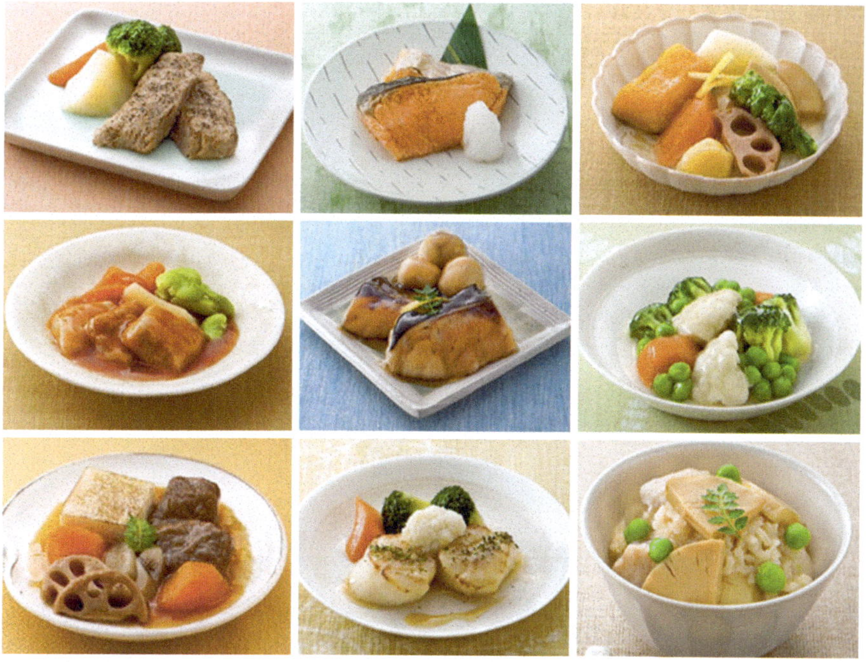

Fig. 7.25 Examples of various types of new modified foods by enzyme homogeneous permeation, namely, iEat products (Reproduced from Otsuka Pharmaceutical Factory, Inc. with permission)

The availability of a wide variety of modified foods in the actual clinical setting allows patients to achieve better outcomes with respect to quality of life and ensures a wide range of foods from which to choose, particularly in the chronic stage of dysphagia.

Thickened Liquids

Thickened liquids have a slower speed of transit through the oral and pharyngeal stages of swallowing. This enhances safe swallowing by allowing better control. Thickening of liquids is widely performed for dysphagic patients, especially those with poor oromotor control of thin liquids in the mouth, a delayed or irregular pharyngeal response, impaired airway protection, and reduced cognitive function because these conditions easily lead to premature spillage, pre-swallowing aspiration, and aspiration during swallowing. Evaluation of the bolus volume is also required to determine whether volume regulation can prevent airway invasion. At FHUR, thickened liquids are classified into three levels of viscosity: thin, nectar, and honey (Table 7.2).

A powdered thickening agent is available for preparation under this classification and is used in both evaluation and swallowing exercise. Many commercial thickeners for liquid modification and/or flavor release in foods containing thickeners are affordable in Japan with relevance to health-related quality-of-life outcomes (Fig. 7.26).

Table 7.2 Classification of thickened liquids corresponding to apparent viscosity (mPa·s) measured at a shear rate of 50 s^{-1}, 20 °C

Category	Bolus	Viscosity (mPa·s)	Viscosity by NDD (centipoises, cP)[a]
Liquid	Thin	16	1–50
	Nectar-like	140	51–350
	Honey-like	460	351–1750

[a]The rightmost column presents the four levels of thickened liquids proposed in the National Dysphagia Diet (1 cP = 1 mPa·s) [43]

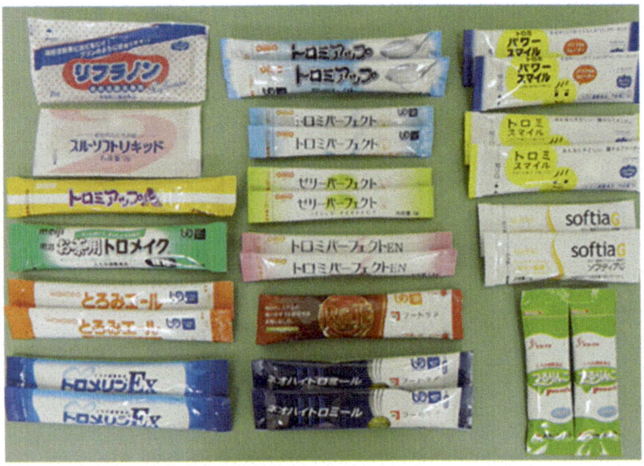

Fig. 7.26 Wide variety of commercial thickening agents available in Japan

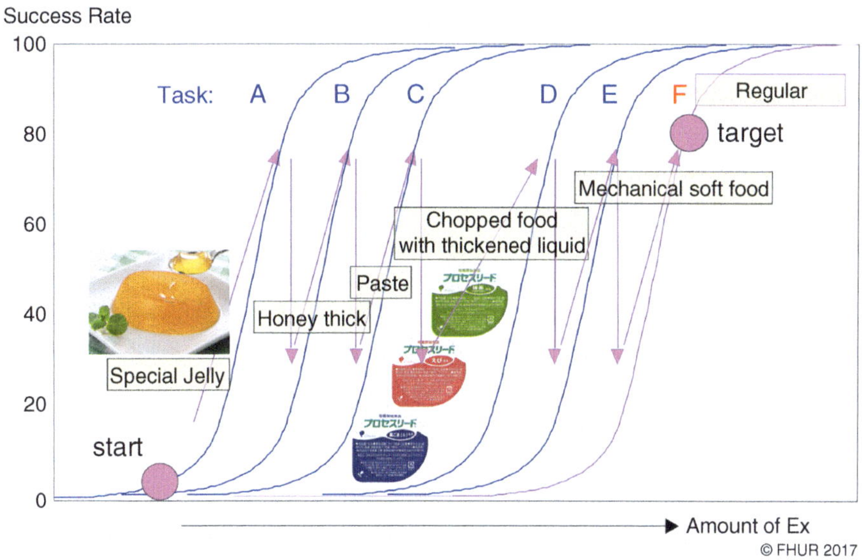

Fig. 7.27 Exercise task with consideration of task difficulty. A stepwise swallowing treatment plan has been formulated in accordance with the motor learning principle

The safety of a texture-modified diet and thickened liquids can be evaluated using VF and VE studies. These investigations should be used to determine whether dysphagic patients will benefit from diet modifications prior to prescription of such diet plans and to determine the adequate level of diet and liquid. When the patients attain the 70% success rate of consumption of current diet and liquid, next level of modified diet and liquid should be provided toward the regular diet. Thus, follow-up of dysphagic patients is needed to reevaluate and adjust the diet to ensure safety and adequate level of difficulty (Fig. 7.27).

The risks of dehydration and malnutrition, which are commonly problematic in dysphagic patients, must be kept in mind. Despite the variety of food modifications available for use, dehydration and malnutrition may still contribute to patients' diminished intake and worsen their nutritional status. Partial dependence on gastrostomy feeding might be necessary for adequate nutrition in patients who have undergone partial restoration of oral intake with an adjusted food consistency. Oral supplements can be added to the regular diets of dysphagic patients to augment their nutritional intake. Likewise, liquid thickening may cause insufficient hydration, necessitating additional water via tube feeding. Dysphagic patients should be frequently evaluated for signs of dehydration and malnutrition. Accordingly, more aggressive nutritional and water support may be warranted.

Appendix

Tongue Range-of-Motion Exercise [6]

Purpose: Improve oral transit (bolus holding, formation, propulsion, and mastication).

Instructions:

1. Extend the tongue straight out of the mouth as far as possible, and then pull the tongue back as far as possible (tongue protrusion exercise).
2. Elevate the back of the tongue as far as possible (tongue retraction exercise).
3. Elevate the tip of the tongue behind the top teeth as high as possible (tongue tip exercise).
4. Move the tongue to each side as far as possible within the oral cavity (tongue lateralization exercise) (Fig. 7.28).

Exercise protocol:

1. Perform and release each exercise 5–10 times; attempt to hold each position for few seconds (up to 6–10 s).
2. Perform three to five sets per day.

Note: Other oral element-based exercises, including range-of-motion exercises of the jaw, cheek muscle-strengthening exercises, and lip closure training, should be considered and concurrently practiced to improve oromotor functional control, particularly with respect to chewing (Fig. 7.29).

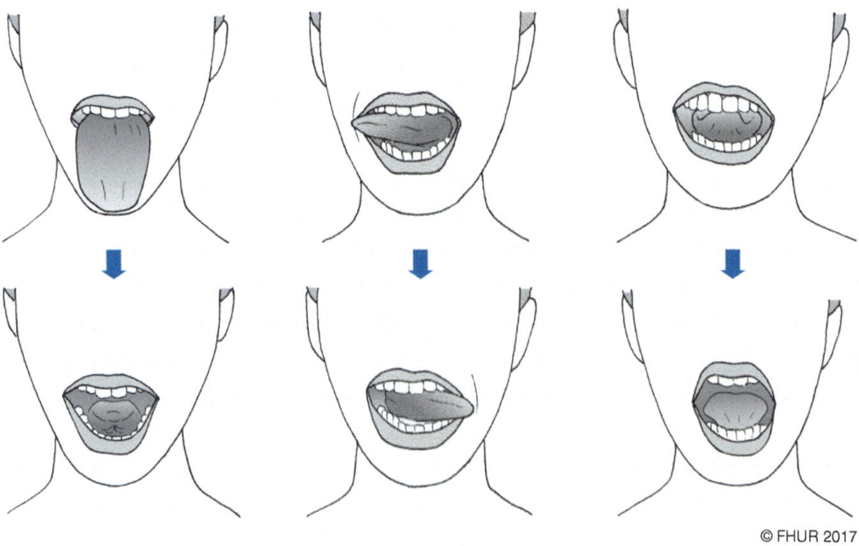

Fig. 7.28 Tongue range-of-motion exercise, (*left*) tongue protrusion-retraction exercise, (*middle*) tongue lateralization exercise, (*right*) tongue elevation exercise (Reproduced from [42] with permission)

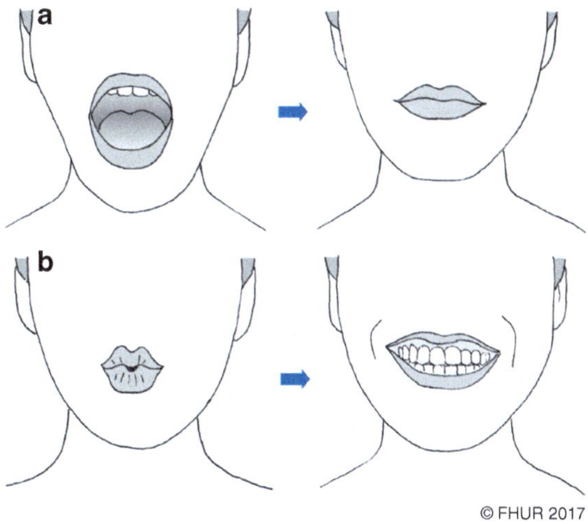

Fig. 7.29 Other oral element-based exercises, (**a**) jaw range-of-motion exercise, (**b**) lip protrusion-retraction exercise (Reproduced from [42] with permission)

Tongue Resistance-Strengthening Exercise

Purpose: Strengthen the tongue to improve oral functions including bolus holding, formation, propulsion, and mastication.

Instructions:

1. Push the tongue against the clinician's finger, tongue depressor, surface of spoon, or Pecopanda*:
   (a) Push the tongue upward against the clinician's finger or Pecopanda* (tongue blade elevation exercise).
   (b) Push the tongue firmly to the left and right sides against a vertical tongue depressor.
   (c) Push the tongue forward firmly against the clinician's finger or tongue depressor.
2. Pull the tongue back with maximum effort against the pulling force provided by the clinician (Fig. 7.30).

Exercise protocol:

1. Hold the pushing or pulling position for a few seconds.
2. Perform each exercise 5–10 times.
3. Perform three to five sets per day.

Note: *The Pecopanda is a tongue-strengthening training tool available at five resistance levels.

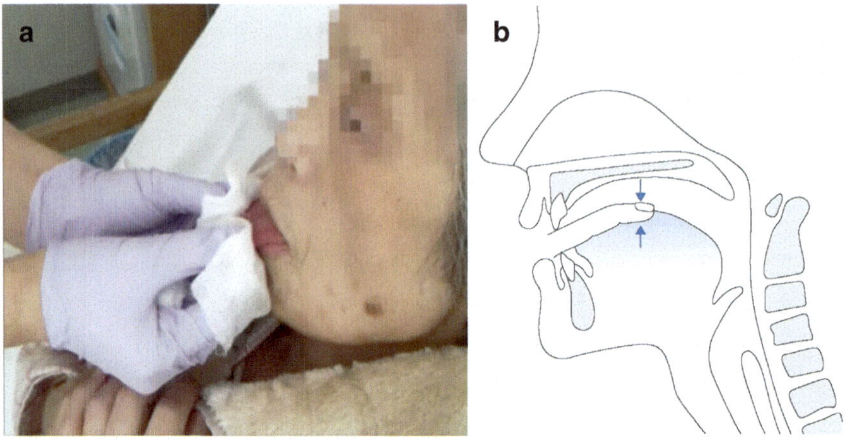

Fig. 7.30 Tongue-strengthening exercises, (**a**) pulling back against the pulling force, (**b**) tongue blade elevation exercise (Reproduced from [42] with permission)

Devices to Facilitate Tongue-Strengthening Exercise

Pecopanda (JMS Co., Ltd., Hiroshima, Japan)

The Pecopanda is a commercialized tool produced by JMS Co. for use with tongue resistance exercises. This tool has five levels of hardness (soft, soft-medium, medium, medium-hard, and hard) depending on the patient's ability. The Pecopanda promotes an understanding of the exercise method and encourages the patient to perform the exercise voluntarily.

Exercise protocol: Recommended frequency is three times a day on more than 3 days per week with a subsequent gradual increase in the exercise load (Figs. 7.31 and 7.32).

Tongue Pressure Measurement Device [4, 40]

A balloon-type tongue pressure measurement device is also produced by JMS Co. This tool is used to measure the tongue pressure and can also be used for incremental strengthening exercises. The device has a digital screen that shows the tongue pressure while the patient performs the exercise and provides a quantitative outcome with which to objectively measure the patient's progression. There is potential to reinforce the patient's exercise performance to achieve the target goal by providing knowledge of his or her performance as feedback; this encourages the patient to achieve a higher pressure and increases patient compliance. The Fujita swallowing team uses this device for isometric progressive resistance oropharyngeal therapy as described below.

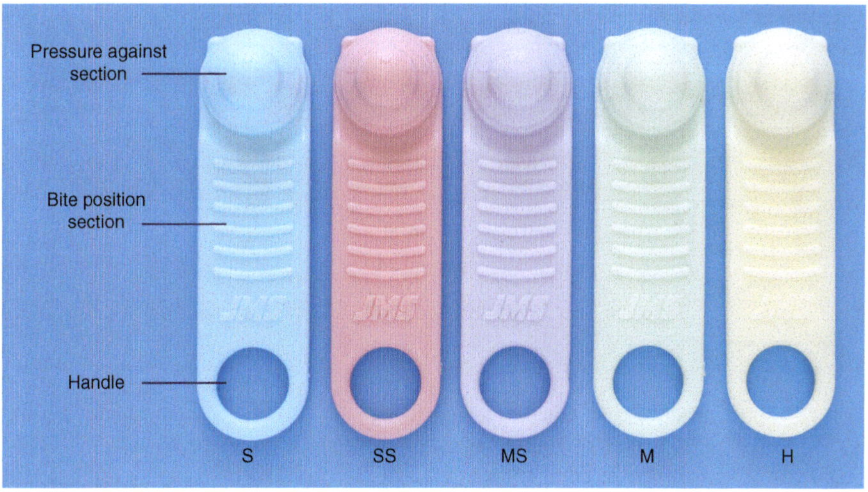

Fig. 7.31 Pecopanda

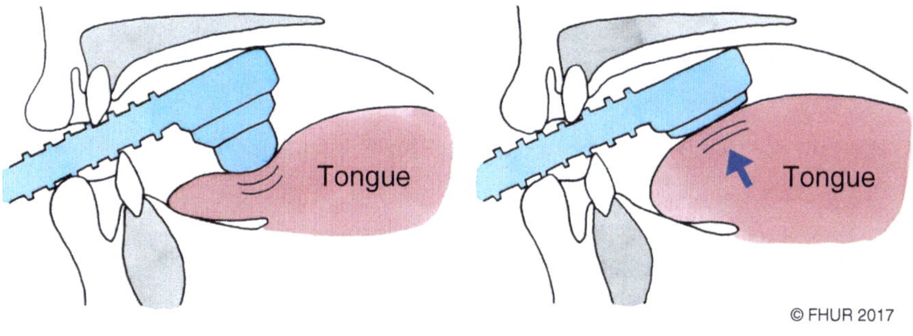

Fig. 7.32 Use of Pecopanda. (*Left*) place the tool between the hard palate and tongue, ensuring stable positioning by fixing the tool using the teeth, and (*right*) push the tongue upward against the tool and hold for a few seconds

Isometric Progressive Resistance Oropharyngeal Therapy

Purpose: Strengthen the tongue to improve oral functions including bolus holding, formation, propulsion, and mastication.

Instructions:

1. Sit in a chair in a relaxed position.
2. Place the balloon (pressure bulb) in the mouth, and hold the plastic pipe at the midpoint of the central incisors with closed lips (Fig. 7.33).
3. Raise the tongue, and firmly compress the balloon onto the hard palate with maximum voluntary effort while counting from 1 to 10. The maximum value is recorded. Perform this exercise six times. The mean of the six measurements is then calculated, representing the baseline maximum tongue pressure.

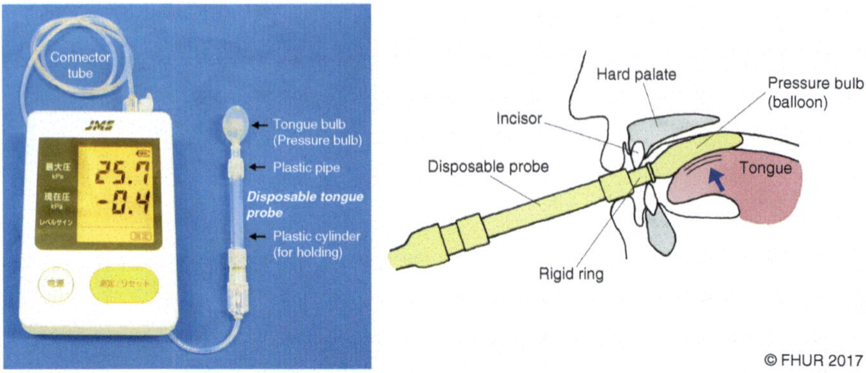

Fig. 7.33 (*Left*) balloon-type tongue pressure device (JMS Co. Ltd., Hiroshima, Japan); (*right*) use of the tongue-strengthening device

Table 7.3 Maximum tongue pressure of healthy subjects in each age group [42]

Age range (year)	Max tongue pressure (kPa)
20–59 (adult male)	45 ± 10
20–59 (adult female)	37 ± 9
Over 60	38 ± 9
Over 70	32 ± 9

4. Perform progressive resistance exercises for 8 weeks, modified from Robbins et al. [41]:
   - First week: 60% of maximum tongue pressure training.
   - Second week: 80% of maximum tongue pressure training.
   - Reevaluate maximum tongue pressure at weeks 3, 5, and 7 to assess clinical improvement and identify progressive changes in exercise target values while practicing at 80% of maximum tongue pressure training.

Exercise protocol: Ten times per set with a 30 s testing interval; three sets per day (this exercise regimen can be modified according to the patient's condition) (Table 7.3).

Oromotor Control Exercise [6]

Purpose: Improve lingual control for bolus manipulation, mastication, and movement.

- Anteroposterior movement of the midline of the tongue during swallow initiation
- Lateralization of the tongue during chewing
- Tongue cupping to hold the bolus
- Tongue elevation against the hard palate

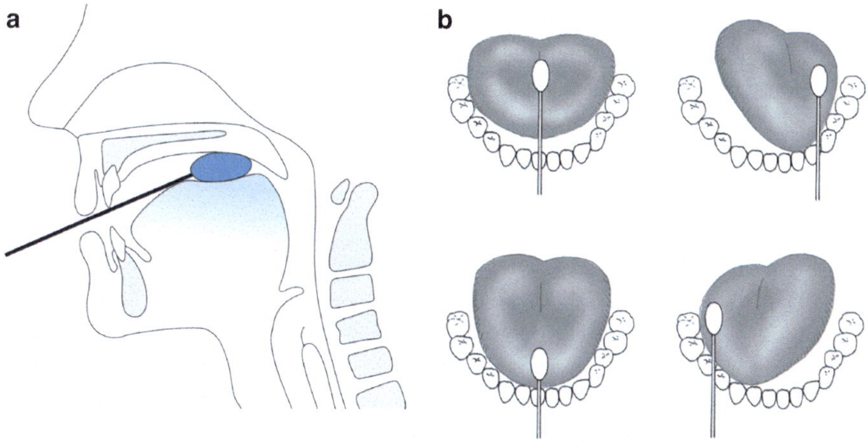

Fig. 7.34 Oromotor control exercise. (**a**) Hold the cotton swab between the tongue and hard palate; (**b**) forward-backward swabbing exercise and lateral swabbing exercise (Reproduced from [42] with permission)

Instructions:

1. Hold a cotton swab between the tongue and hard palate.
2. Move it from one side to the other, and then slide it forward and backward.
3. Move it in a circular fashion from the middle of the tongue to the teeth on one side, back to the middle of the tongue, and then to the opposite side of the teeth in the same manner; this constitutes one cycle (Fig. 7.34).

Exercise protocol:

1. Move in each direction 5–10 times.
2. Perform three to five sets per day.
3. Gradually increase the speed of the movements.

Shaker Exercise [2]

Purpose: Improve hyolaryngeal superoanterior movement by physiologically strengthening the suprahyoid muscles (including the digastric, mylohyoid, geniohyoid muscles), thus improving UES opening.

Instructions: Lie in the supine position with no pillow under the head, and then perform the following two-part exercise:

Part 1: Isometric component

- One minute sustained head raise, repeat three times with 1 min rest between repetitions.

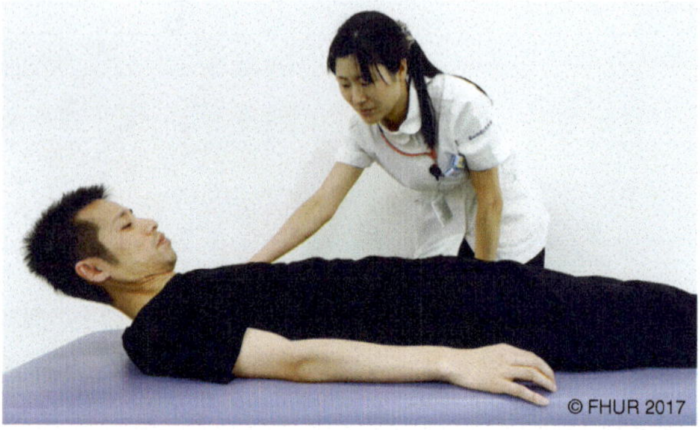

Fig. 7.35 Shaker exercise. The head is raised off of the floor or bed to look at the toes without raising the shoulders

Part 2: Isokinetic component

- Thirty consecutive repetitions of head raise (without rest) (Fig. 7.35)

Exercise protocol: Perform three times per day, 7 days per week for 6 weeks.
Notes:

- The patient is instructed to lift the head to look at the toes or umbilicus while keeping the shoulders flat on the floor or bed and continuing to breathe while performing the exercise.
- If the patient is too weak to complete the exercise protocol, the regimen should be adjusted on an individual basis to improve endurance.

Limitations: tracheostomy tube placement, limited neck mobility, and cervical spine deficits

Jaw-Opening Exercise [5]

Purpose: Improve UES opening during the swallow.
Instructions:

1. Maximally open the jaw and maintain for 10 s with a 10 s rest in between each exercise.
2. Attempt to strongly contract the suprahyoid muscles during the exercise.
3. Repeat five times.

Exercise protocol: Perform two sets of five repetitions daily for 4 weeks.
Note: Caution is needed in patients with a history of mandibular arthritis, degeneration of the articular disk of the temporomandibular joint, or temporomandibular joint dislocation.

Tongue Base Retraction Exercise

Purpose: Improve tongue base retraction strength to better propel the bolus and increase pharyngeal pressure.

Instructions:

1. Pull the back of the tongue (tongue base) as far back into the mouth as possible and hold it for a few seconds.
2. Pull the back of the tongue (tongue base) as far back into the mouth as possible, pretend to gargle hard, and then release.
3. Yawn while pulling the tongue as far back as possible, and hold the mouth open as wide as possible for 1–2 s.

Exercise protocol: Perform three times per day, 7 days per week for 6 weeks.

Tongue-Holding Swallow Exercise (Masako Maneuver)

Purpose: Improve posterior pharyngeal muscle contraction.

Instructions:

1. Protrude the tongue from the mouth.
2. Hold the anterior portion of the tongue gently between the front teeth or gums.
3. Swallow while keeping the tongue protruded (Fig. 7.36).

Exercise protocol: Perform the exercise 10 times per set and 1–2 sets per day.

Note: This maneuver must be practiced only with saliva swallowing while incrementally increasing the range of protrusion.

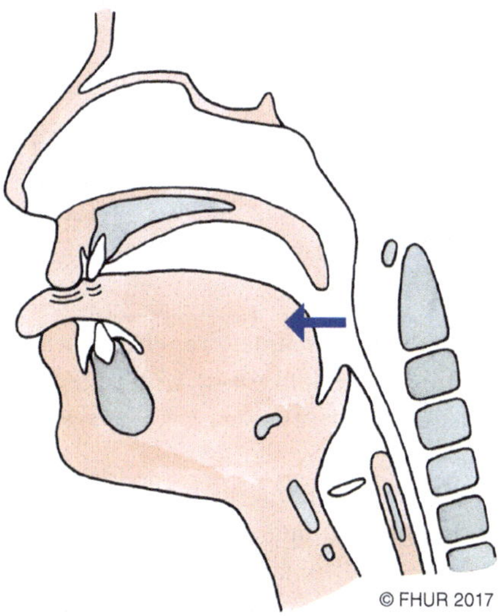

Fig. 7.36 Illustration of tongue protrusion during the Masako (tongue-hold) maneuver

Expiratory Muscle-Strengthening Exercise

Purpose: Breathe out against resistance (positive pressure) to gain expiratory muscle strength with the added benefit of vibrations (oscillations) to clear secretions.

Device 1: Acapella®

The Acapella® is a handheld airway clearance device that combines the resistance of a positive expiratory pressure device with a vibratory mode for airway clearance.

Two devices, distinguished by color, are available:

- Green or high-flow device: for patients who are able to maintain an expiratory flow of ≥15 L/min for 3 s. The green Acapella is suitable for most patients.
- Blue or low-flow device: for patients with low peak expiratory flow of <15 L/min for 3 s. The blue Acapella is commonly used in children and older patients.

Exercise protocol:

- The maximum expiratory pressure (MEP) is measured in each patient to determine the resistance level during training.
- Generally start with the resistance set at 30% of the MEP and inspiratory: expiratory ratio at 1:3–1:4.
- Perform the exercise 10–20 times per set and 1–4 sets per day (the exercise program can be adjusted depending on the patient's condition).
- Reevaluate weekly to adjust the level of resistance until reaching 60–80% of the MEP.

Device 2: Threshold Positive Expiratory Pressure Device (Threshold PEP™)

The Threshold PEP™ is a flow-dependent, one-way valve threshold device that is used to maintain constant pressure regardless of the patient's airflow. Therefore, a pressure indicator is unnecessary. This device can be used with a mouthpiece or mask for increased ease of use.

Instructions:

- The patient maintains a relaxed or comfortable sitting position.
- Hold the patient's nose with a nose clip as necessary. Breathe through the mouth.
- The MEP is measured in each patient to determine the resistance level during training.
- Placing mouthpiece device between the lips and behind the teeth. Seal lips around mouthpiece.
- Take a full inhale and then exhale 3–4 times longer than inhale. Continue this pattern during training as recommended in an exercise protocol.

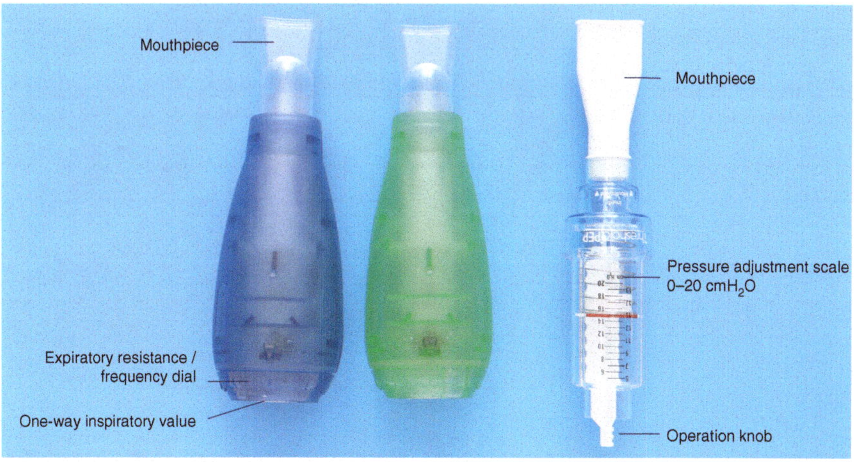

Fig. 7.37 Handheld airway clearance devices, (**a**) Acapella®, (**b**) Threshold PEP™

Exercise protocol:

- The therapist sets the level of resistance at 30% of the MEP at the beginning of training and sets the inspiratory/expiratory ratio at 1:3–1:4.
- The resistance measurement will be reset weekly (adjusted depending on the patient's condition).
- The exercise is performed for 10–20 min per set (5–10 times per set), and 2–4 sets are performed per day for 4 weeks (Fig. 7.37).

Notable issues:

- Focus on slow and prolonged exhalation following the inspiratory phase.
- Neither device is gravity-dependent and can be used in any position nor in conjunction with postural drainage.

Thermal-Tactile Stimulation

Purpose: Decrease the threshold of the pharyngeal swallow response and improve the triggering speed of the pharyngeal swallow.

Techniques:

1. Place a cold, wet cotton swab in contact with the anterior faucial arches, and maintain this position while vertically rubbing it up and down.
2. Complete five strokes along each arch followed by a saliva swallow.

Exercise protocol: Perform once to twice daily (Fig. 7.38).

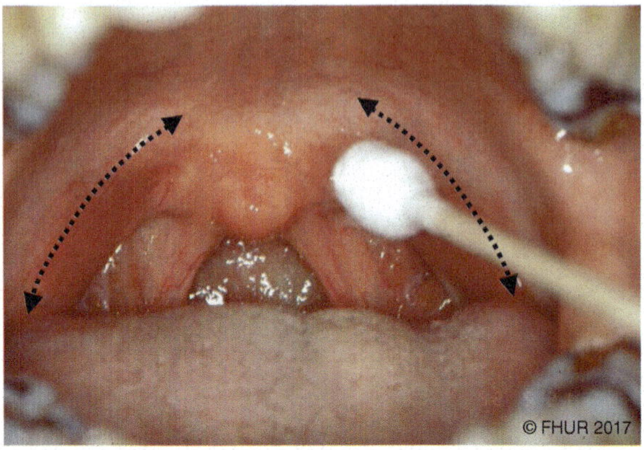

Fig. 7.38 Placement of cold, wet cotton swab at the anterior faucial arches, where thermal-tactile stimulation is to occur

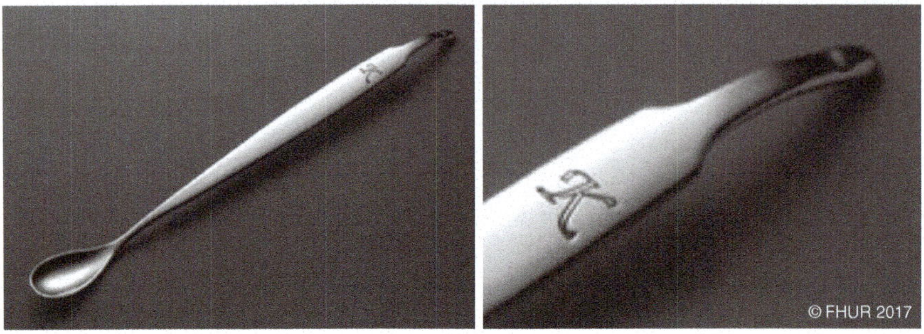

Fig. 7.39 (*Left*) K-Spoon, (*right*) tip of K-Spoon used for K-point stimulation

K-Spoon

The K-Spoon (Aoyoshi Co., Ltd., Niigata, Japan) was invented by Kojima for concomitant use with K-point stimulation; it can be employed for other purposes as well. This tool is lightweight, of adequate length, thin, and easy to hold during swallowing training. In addition, it is easy to control the bolus volume (2 ml) during direct training. The K-Spoon is made of metal, and the tip on the side opposite that for holding food can be easily used for cold stimulation at the K-point (Fig. 7.39).

Balloon Dilatation

Purpose: Gain temporary flexibility and expand the luminal diameter of the UES, particularly used in patients with cricopharyngeal dysfunction (e.g., supratentorial lesion, brain stem stroke) and disuse syndrome.

Inclusion criteria:

1. Patients with a large amount of pharyngeal residue after swallowing without evidence of UES opening on VF or VE study.
2. No structural abnormality of the pharynx or larynx.
3. No mass effect originating from outside, such as that induced by a tumor.
4. No strong gag reflex during balloon insertion.
5. Failure of other compensatory strategies.
6. Patient is cooperative during the procedure.

Methods:

1. Check the condition of the balloon catheter; a 12- to 14-Fr urethral catheter is typically used.
2. Mark the catheter surface at 1 cm intervals, beginning approximately 20 cm from the catheter end. These marks correspond to the mouth angle when the dilated balloon is presented at the UES during VF.
3. Insert barium solution through the catheter for visualization on VF.
4. Typically, the catheter is transorally inserted (in patients with a high level of gag reflex sensitization; however, transnasal insertion is performed instead). Stop when the catheter tip passes through the UES. The position of the balloon catheter in the esophagus is confirmed on the VF image.
5. Inflate the balloon with 2–3 ml of air, and then pull the catheter backward until resistance against the pulling force is felt.
6. Record the marker seen on the catheter at the front teeth or the mouth angle as the position of the lower margin of the UES. This marker is helpful to maintain the position of the catheter during dilatation.
7. Perform balloon dilatation. Four balloon-expanding techniques are used in Japan:

   A. Intermittent dilatation method

   After resistance is felt as mentioned in Step 5, slightly deflate the catheter and move it <1 cm proximally; thus, the balloon is positioned at the level of the UES. Slowly inflate air into the balloon and increase the volume in 0.5–1.0 ml increments based on the patient's tolerance. Try to sustain the dilatation for several seconds (up to 10 s) at the same position until the catheter passes through the UES.

   B. Pulling with simultaneous swallowing

   After resistance is felt as mentioned in Step 5, pull the balloon through the UES while instructing the patient to swallow the balloon.

   C. Pulling without simultaneous swallowing

   After resistance is felt as mentioned in Step 5, simply pull the balloon without instructing the patient to swallow it (in techniques B and C, the balloon size can be gradually increased as tolerated by the patient to a maximum of 10 ml).

D. Balloon swallowing method

Insert the balloon catheter into the lower pharynx and inflate it to 1.0–1.5 ml. Ask the patient to swallow with effort to pass the balloon through the UES. The catheter can be pushed slightly while the patient swallows.

Balloon dilatation is performed repeatedly three times on the impaired side to evaluate the immediate effect. In patients with bilateral lesions, the execution of this therapeutic procedure is recommended to be first performed on less severely affected side. Techniques B and C are easily performed by the patient or the patient's caregivers.

Exercise protocol: Perform 5–10 times per session on each side of the UES, 1–3 sessions per day, and 5–7 days per week for 1–3 consecutive months.

Notes:

- At FHUR, the intermittent dilatation method is used under VF guidance by confirming the location of the balloon; however, the pulling method either with or without simultaneous swallowing is used during training because of the possibility of self-performance.
- In our experience, no dilatation-related complications such as pain, bleeding, tissue injury, or vagovagal reflex-related shock have occurred.

Supraglottic and Super-Supraglottic Swallow

Supraglottic Swallow

Kinesiology: Increase true vocal fold closure and arytenoid medial approximation before and during swallowing.

Effect: Enhance airway protection

Instructions:

1. Breathe in deeply.
2. Hold breath.
3. Swallow while maintaining the breath hold.
4. Cough immediately, and then swallow again before breathing (Fig. 7.40).

Super-Supraglottic Swallow

Kinesiology: Mainly increase closure of all laryngeal structures before and during swallowing; also increase base of tongue retraction, pressure generation, and earlier and prolonged UES opening.

Effects: Greater airway protection and enhanced pharyngeal clearance

Instructions:

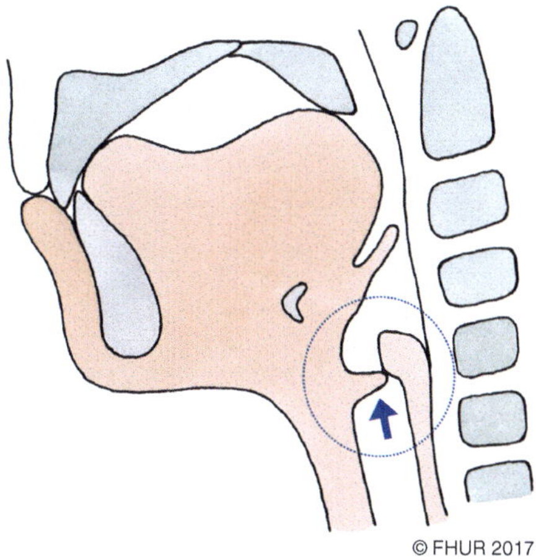

Fig. 7.40 Effect of supraglottic swallow

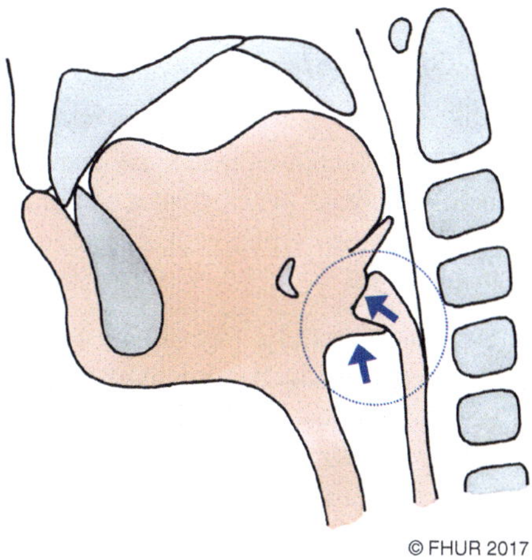

Fig. 7.41 Effect of super-supraglottic swallow

1. Take a deep breath and hold it very tightly while bearing down.
2. Swallow hard while maintaining the tight breath hold.
3. Cough immediately after this swallow; then immediately swallow hard again before breathing (Fig. 7.41).

   Notes:

- In both the supraglottic and super-supraglottic swallowing maneuvers, VE and VF studies are used for visual performance feedback to determine whether the TVCs are properly closed and maintained while swallowing.
- For dysphagic patients with problematic TVC closure, simply holding the breath may more effectively achieve TVC closure than the combination of taking a deep breath and then holding the breath. This could be because a deep breath widens (abducts) the TVCs, and they are difficult to close afterward [21].

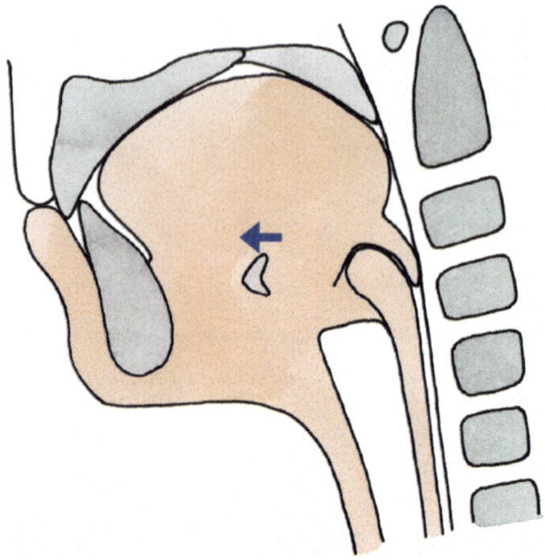

Fig. 7.42 Effect of Mendelsohn maneuver

Mendelsohn Maneuver

Kinesiology: Increase the extension and duration of hyolaryngeal elevation and subsequently increase the extension and duration of UES opening.

Effects: Improve pharyngeal clearance capability and swallow coordination.

Instructions:

1. Swallow normally. Pay attention to and feel elevation of the larynx (Adam's apple) during swallowing by palpating its upward movement with the index finger and thumb.
2. When the Adam's apple reaches the highest point of elevation, attempt to hold it with the throat muscles for several seconds, and then complete the swallow (Fig. 7.42).

Effortful Swallow [26, 27]

Kinesiology: Increase tongue base retraction and pressure during pharyngeal swallowing.

Effect: Improve capability of bolus clearance, particularly in the vallecula

Instructions:

1. Swallow really hard, squeezing your throat muscles forcefully.
2. Pretend like you have a big piece of steak or bagel in the mouth, and it's tough to pass down—you need to put a lot of effort into it (Fig. 7.43).

Fig. 7.43 Effect of effortful swallow

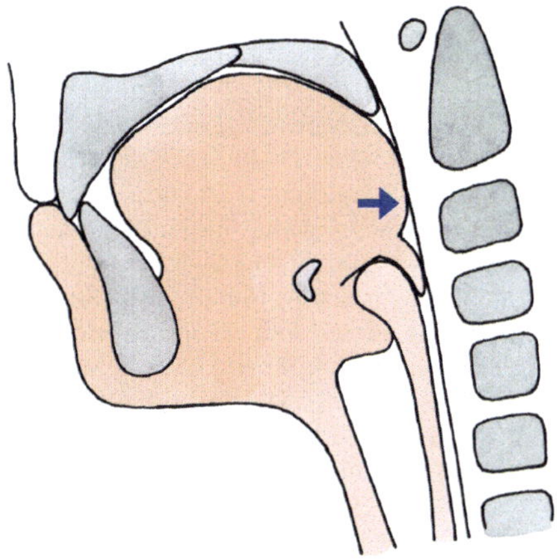

References

1. Schmidt RA. Motor learning & performance: from principles to practice. 1st ed. Champaign: Human Kinetics; 1991.
2. Shaker R, Kern M, Bardan E, Taylor A, Stewart ET, Hoffmann RG, et al. Augmentation of deglutitive upper esophageal sphincter opening in the elderly by exercise. Am J Physiol Gastrointest Liver Physiol. 1997;272(6):G1518–22.
3. Shaker R, Easterling C, Kern M, Nitschke T, Massey B, Daniels S, et al. Rehabilitation of swallowing by exercise in tube-fed patients with pharyngeal dysphagia secondary to abnormal UES opening. Gastroenterology. 2002;122(5):1314–21.
4. Utanohara Y, Hayashi R, Yoshikawa M, Yoshida M, Tsuga K, Akagawa Y. Standard values of maximum tongue pressure taken using newly developed disposable tongue pressure measurement device. Dysphagia. 2008;23(3):286–90. doi:10.1007/s00455-007-9142-z.
5. Wada S, Tohara H, Iida T, Inoue M, Sato M, Ueda K. Jaw-opening exercise for insufficient opening of upper esophageal sphincter. Arch Phys Med Rehabil. 2012;93(11):1995–9. doi:10.1016/j.apmr.2012.04.025.
6. Logemann JA. Evaluation and treatment of swallowing disorders. 2nd ed. Austin (TX): Pro-Ed; 1998.
7. Fujiu M, Logemann JA, Pauloski BR. Increased postoperative posterior pharyngeal wall movement in patients with anterior oral cancer: preliminary findings and possible implications for treatment. Am J Speech Lang Pathol. 1995;4(2):24–30. doi:10.1044/1058-0360.0402.24.
8. Fujiu M, Logemann JA. Effect of a tongue-holding maneuver on posterior pharyngeal wall movement during deglutition. Am J Speech Lang Pathol. 1996;5(1):23–30. doi:10.1044/1058-0360.0501.23.
9. Fujiu-Kurachi M. Symposium: EBM of the tongue-holding maneuver. Jpn J Speech Lang Hear Res. 2010;7(1):31–8. (Japanese)
10. Fujiu-Kurachi M. Developing the tongue holding maneuver. Dysphagia. 2002;11(1):9–11. doi:10.1044/sasd11.1.9.
11. Pitts T, Bolser D, Rosenbek J, Troche M, Okun MS, Sapienza C. Impact of expiratory muscle strength training on voluntary cough and swallow function in Parkinson disease. Chest. 2009;135(5):1301–8. doi:10.1378/chest.08-1389.

12. Troche MS, Okun MS, Rosenbek JC, Musson N, Fernandez HH, Rodriguez R, et al. Aspiration and swallowing in Parkinson disease and rehabilitation with EMST: a randomized trial. Neurology. 2010;75(21):1912–9. doi:10.1212/WNL.0b013e3181fef115.
13. Lazzara GL, Lazarus CL, Logemann JA. Impact of thermal stimulation on the triggering of the swallowing reflex. Dysphagia. 1986;1(2):73–7. doi:10.1007/BF02407117.
14. Kojima C, Fujishima I, Ohkuma R, Maeda H, Shibamoto I, Hojo K, et al. Jaw opening and swallow triggering method for bilateral-brain-damaged patients: K-point stimulation. Dysphagia. 2002;17(4):273–7.
15. Sumiya N, Ishida A, Murakami K. Rehabilitation of pharyngeal dysphagia: intermittent air stretching method with balloon catheter. Jpn J Rehabil Med. 1997;34(8):553–9. (Japanese)
16. Onogi K, Saitoh E, Kondo I, Ozeki M, Kagaya H. Immediate effectiveness of balloon dilatation therapy for patients with dysphagia due to cricopharyngeal dysfunction. Jpn J Compr Rehabil Sci. 2014;5:87–92.
17. Hojo K, Fujishima I, Ohno T, Kojima C, Takehara I, Sibamoto I, et al. Research into the effectiveness how well the balloon dilatation method causes the desired outcome for cricopharyngeal dysphagia at the chronic stage in cerebrovascular disease. Jpn J Speech Lang Heari Res. 2006;3:106–15.
18. Martin BJ, Logemann JA, Shaker R, Dodds WJ. Normal laryngeal valving patterns during three breath-hold maneuvers: a pilot investigation. Dysphagia. 1993;8(1):11–20.
19. Ohmae Y, Logemann JA, Kaiser P, Hanson DG, Kahrilas PJ. Effects of two breath-holding maneuvers on oropharyngeal swallow. Ann Otol Rhinol Laryngol. 1996;105(2):123–31.
20. Logemann JA, Pauloski BR, Rademaker AW, Colangelo LA. Super-supraglottic swallow in irradiated head and neck cancer patients. Head Neck. 1997;19(6):535–40.
21. Donzelli J, Brady S. The effects of breath-holding on vocal fold adduction: implications for safe swallowing. Arch Otolaryngol Head Neck Surg. 2004;130(2):208–10.
22. Kahrilas PJ, Logemann JA, Krugler C, Flanagan E. Volitional augmentation of upper esophageal sphincter opening during swallowing. Am J Phys. 1991;260(3 Pt 1):G450–6.
23. Mendelsohn MS, McConnel FM. Function in the pharyngoesophageal segment. Laryngoscope. 1987;97(4):483–9.
24. McCullough GH, Kim Y. Effects of the Mendelsohn maneuver on extent of hyoid movement and UES opening post-stroke. Dysphagia. 2013;28(4):511–9. doi:10.1007/s00455-013-9461-1.
25. Lazarus C, Logemann JA, Gibbons P. Effects of maneuvers on swallowing function in a dysphagic oral cancer patient. Head Neck. 1993;15(5):419–24.
26. Lazarus CL, Logemann JA, Song CW, Rademaker AW, Kahrilas PJ. Effects of voluntary maneuvers on tongue base function for swallowing. Folia Phoniatr Logop. 2002;54:171–6.
27. Karle WE, Lazarus CL. Swallowing rehabilitation. In: Fried M, Tan M, editors. Laryngology for the general otolaryngologist. New York: Thieme; 2014.
28. Pouderoux P, Kahrilas PJ. Deglutitive tongue force modulation by volition, volume, and viscosity in humans. Gastroenterology. 1995;108(5):1418–26.
29. Hind JA, Nicosia MA, Roecker EB, Carnes ML, Robbins J. Comparison of effortful and noneffortful swallows in healthy middle-aged and older adults. Arch Phys Med Rehabil. 2001;82(12):1661–5.
30. Huckabee ML, Butler SG, Barclay M, Jit S. Submental surface electromyographic measurement and pharyngeal pressures during normal and effortful swallowing. Arch Phys Med Rehabil. 2005;86(11):2144–9.
31. Kagaya H, Inamoto Y, Okada S, Saitoh E. Body positions and functional training to reduce aspiration in patients with dysphagia. JMAJ. 2011;54(1):35–8.
32. Saitoh E, Kimura A, Yamori S, Mori H, Izumi S, Chino N. Videofluorography in rehabilitation of dysphagia. Jpn J Rehabil Med. 1986;23(3):121–4. (Japanese)
33. Logemann JA, Kahrilas PJ, Kobara M, Vakil NB. The benefit of head rotation on pharyngoesophageal dysphagia. Arch Phys Med Rehabil. 1989;70(10):767–71.
34. Ohmae Y, Ogura M, Kitahara S, Karaho T, Inouye T. Effects of head rotation on pharyngeal function during normal swallow. Ann Otol Rhinol Laryngol. 1998;107(4):344–8.

35. Inamoto Y, Saitoh E, Shibata S, Kagaya H, Nakayama E, Ota K, et al. Effectiveness and applicability of a specialized evaluation exercise-chair in posture adjustment for swallowing. Jpn J Compr Rehabil Sci. 2014;5:33–9.
36. Okada S, Saitoh E, Palmer JB, Matsuo K, Yokoyama M, Shigeta R, et al. What is the chin-down posture? A questionnaire survey of speech language pathologists in Japan and the United States. Dysphagia. 2007;22(3):204–9.
37. Yokoyama M, Okada S, Baba M, Saitoh E, Shigeta R, Suzuki M, et al. A new jelly-type food for dysphagia patients–study on its usage in direct therapy. Jpn J Dysphagia Rehabil. 2005;9:186–94. (Japanese)
38. Nakagawa K, Matsuo K, Shibata S, Inamoto Y, Ito Y, Abe K, et al. Efficacy of a novel training food based on the process model of feeding for mastication and swallowing——a preliminary study in elderly individuals living at a residential facility. Jpn J Compr Rehabil Sci. 2014;5:72–8.
39. Umene S, Hayashi M, Kato K, Masunaga H. Physical properties of root crops treated with novel softening technology capable of retaining the shape, color, and nutritional value of foods. Dysphagia. 2015;30(2):105–13. doi:10.1007/s00455-014-9581-2.
40. Aoki Y, Kabuto S, Ozeki Y, Tanaka T, Ota K. The effect of tongue pressure strengthening exercise for dysphagic patients. Jpn J Compr Rehabil Sci. 2015;6:129–36.
41. Robbins J, Kays SA, Gangnon RE, Hind JA, Hewitt AL, Gentry LR, et al. The effects of lingual exercise in stroke patients with dysphagia. Arch Phys Med Rehabil. 2007;88(2):150–8.
42. Dysphagia Team of Seirei; Fujishima I, supervised. Pocket manual of dysphagia. 3rd ed. Tokyo: Ishiyaku Publications Inc; 2011. (Japanese)
43. Cichero JA, Steele C, Duivestein J, Clavé P, Chen J, Kayashita J, et al. The need for international terminology and definitions for texture-modified foods and thickened liquids used in dysphagia management: foundations of a global initiative. Curr Phys Med Rehabil Rep. 2013;1:280–91.

Chapter 8
Other Swallowing Treatments

Yoko Inamoto, Kannit Pongpipatpaiboon, Seiko Shibata, Yoichiro Aoyagai, Hitoshi Kagaya, and Koichiro Matsuo

Abstract In addition to several methods of swallowing exercise widely used to improve swallowing function, the alternative treatment by using assistive device and surgical intervention are viable options to achieve the treatment outcome, for safety and for improved quality of life. The common devices and surgical techniques commonly used in our practice are described in this chapter.

8.1 Assistive System

8.1.1 Intermittent Oral Catheterization

Intermittent oral catheterization was developed in Japan as an alternative nutritional management technique in dysphagic patients [1, 2]. This technique protects against aspiration pneumonia and counters malnutrition both in patients with difficulty ingesting a sufficient amount of food and in those with no oral intake ability [2, 3]. The patient inserts a feeding tube into his or her mouth (or nose if the gag reflex is hypersensitive) until the tip reaches the mid-esophagus, and the tube is promptly removed when infusion of the meal has finished. Before using this method, esophageal function should be investigated by VF study. In patients with esophageal peristaltic dysfunction, the tip of the tube should be placed in the stomach rather than the mid-esophagus (Fig. 8.1).

Y. Inamoto (✉)
Faculty of Rehabilitation, School of Health Sciences, Fujita Health University, Toyoake, Aichi, Japan
e-mail: inamoto@fujita-hu.ac.jp

K. Pongpipatpaiboon • S. Shibata • Y. Aoyagai • H. Kagaya
Department of Rehabilitation Medicine I, School of Medicine, Fujita Health University, Toyoake, Aichi, Japan
e-mail: ning665@gmail.com; sshibata@fujita-hu.ac.jp; yyy@rc5.so-net.ne.jp; hkagaya2@fujita-hu.ac.jp

K. Matsuo
Department of Dentistry, School of Medicine, Fujita Health University, Toyoake, Aichi, Japan
e-mail: kmatsuo@fujita-hu.ac.jp

E. Saitoh et al. (eds.), *Dysphagia Evaluation and Treatment*,
https://doi.org/10.1007/978-981-10-5032-9_8

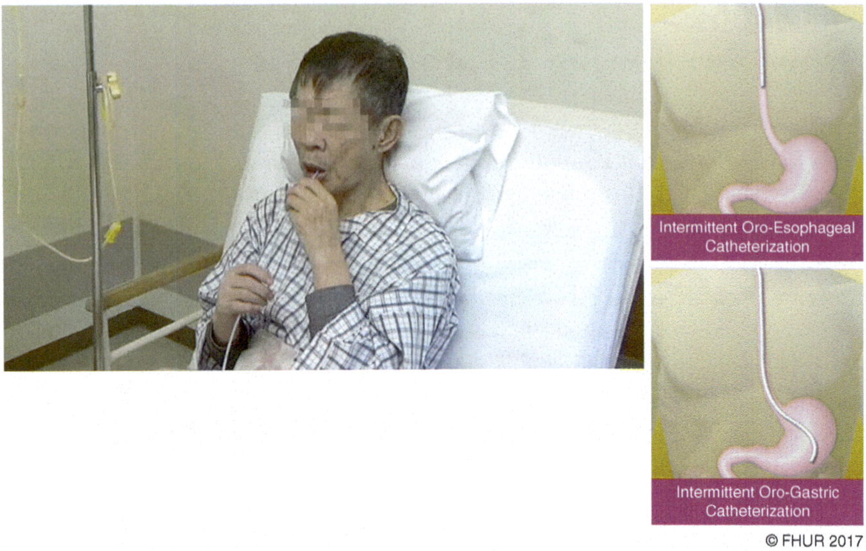

Fig. 8.1 Intermittent oral self-catheterization. Two locations of the catheter tip are possible depending on the patient's condition

The recommended feeding speed is usually 150–200 ml/h when placing the catheter tip in the stomach to prevent vomiting [4]. If the catheter tip is placed along the esophageal route, the feeding speed can be higher due to physiological enteric mobility, which is triggered following esophageal peristalsis. The patient should be instructed to intentionally swallow saliva during tube feeding to promote esophageal peristalsis and prevent gastroesophageal regurgitation.

Intermittent oral catheterization can be a method of swallowing treatment. Swallowing is more likely to be triggered with tube than saliva swallowing. Therefore, swallowing the tube at every feeding (three times/day) intermittently provides the increase of swallowing frequency. Additionally, it helps to prevent the decrease of sensation, which is caused by long-term tube placement. The social benefits of intermittent oral catheterization include the aesthetic appearance without tube.

8.1.2 Dental Prostheses

In addition to oral hygiene care, dentists are responsible for prosthetic management of swallowing disorders, i.e., oral prosthodontics. A dental prosthesis is an intraoral prosthesis used to restore (reconstruct) intraoral defects and thus improve morphological swallowing function. It acts as an auxiliary device for treatment of oral functional abnormalities primarily related to postoperative oral cancer, maxillofacial trauma, or neurologic/motor deficits with tongue paralysis. Various types of oral prostheses are designed to improve the oral stage of swallowing, such as the palatal augmentation prosthesis, palatal lift prosthesis, and lingual augmentation prosthesis

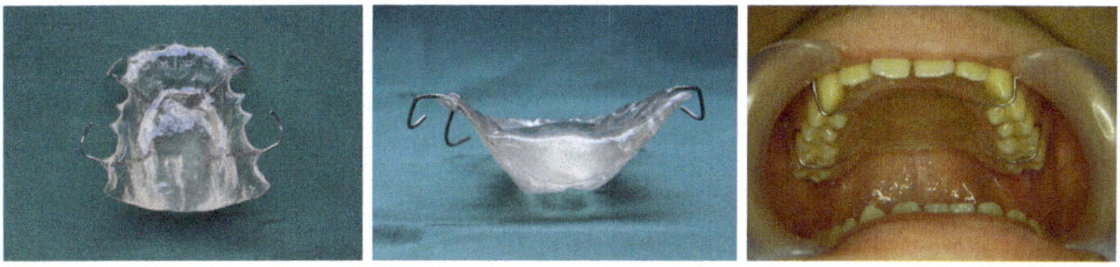

Fig. 8.2 Palatal augmentation prosthesis: the most common oral prosthesis for enhancing swallowing ability

[5–8]. The advantages of these prostheses include improved chewing, accommodation for bolus formation and control in the mouth, a decreased tongue–palate distance, and increased propulsive pressure for bolus transit. Like other swallowing treatments, the efficacy of prostheses can be determined by VF study, ensuring the best functional outcome.

The palatal augmentation prosthesis is one of the most common oral prostheses used in dysphagic patients with tongue movement disorders caused by postoperative tongue resection due to cancer, amyotrophic lateral sclerosis, stroke, and other conditions (Fig. 8.2). The morphological mechanism of the palatal augmentation prosthesis involves a decrease in the volume of the oral cavity by establishment of a lower palatal vault level; thus, less tongue bulk and motility are required to transport the bolus to the posterior oral cavity, and the tongue–palate contact pressure increases to propel the bolus into the oropharynx. The effectiveness of the palatal augmentation prosthesis for swallowing is provided by the improvement in the tongue pressure and tongue base pressure, which leads to [9–11]:

- A shortened oral transit time
- A shortened pharyngeal transit time
- Facilitation of contact between the base of the tongue and posterior pharyngeal wall
- Improved articulation

8.2 Surgical Treatment

Severe dysphagia with intractable aspiration is a life-threatening medical condition. Surgical intervention should be considered if extensive swallowing rehabilitation has failed. At FHUR, otolaryngologists collaborate with a transdisciplinary swallowing team and play a major role in the specific reconstructive surgery performed for such patients: a particular combination of bilateral cricopharyngeal myotomy (or UES myotomy) and laryngeal suspension.

Various surgical procedures have been described to treat chronic aspiration and recurrent pneumonia in patients with severe dysphagia (e.g., total laryngectomy, laryngeal closure, and laryngeal diversion) [12, 13]. Most procedures involve the creation of a permanent tracheostoma and result in loss of normal phonation. UES myotomy and laryngeal suspension were alternatively developed for preservation of normal phonation and respiration without a permanent tracheostomy, as described in the next section. The goal of this surgery is to prevent life-threatening aspiration [13–16] with preservation of a functional larynx and facilitation of oral nutrition; this procedure is not used to normalize the swallowing function (Appendix "UES Myotomy Combined with Laryngeal Suspension").

Temporary tracheostomy is routinely performed in the postoperative period to protect the airway in case of airway compromise and the need for intubation. A narrower laryngeal entrance caused by laryngeal suspension and/or edema could result in dyspnea. Tracheostomy is also important to ensure the safety of performing swallowing exercises. It is imperative to ensure that the patients and their families understand that several months of postoperative dysphagia rehabilitation is necessary to augment oropharyngeal muscle strengthening and perform exercises for the new swallowing pattern.

The specific postoperative training exercise for the new swallow pattern is a combination of head extension and neck flexion for opening the UES (chin jut).

Patients must learn to perform this posture performance on the right time when the bolus reaches the pharynx. While giving visual feedback to patients, VE is often utilized to ensure that patients achieve an accurate sense of the degrees and timing of head extension and neck flexion. Simultaneously extending the head and flexing the neck moves the mandible and larynx anterosuperiorly, which consequently opens the esophageal inlet (Fig. 8.3).

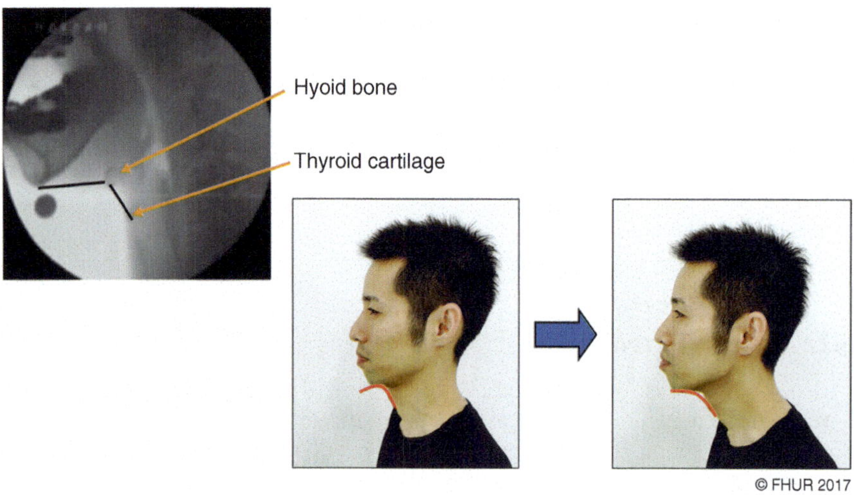

Fig. 8.3 The new swallowing pattern involves head extension and neck flexion to augment opening of the UES entrance. Lateral fluoroscopic views show that the bolus has easily passed through the widening of the esophageal inlet while performing head extension and neck flexion after UES myotomy combined with laryngeal suspension

Dysphagia rehabilitation is required for several months postoperatively. If bolus propulsion with respect to tongue function is preserved/improved and aspiration is successfully prevented, oral intake up to the level of a regular diet can be expected. In contrary, when aspiration and pharyngeal residue cannot be eliminated despite the performance of postoperative rehabilitation, oral intake will be restricted to a paste-type food or nothing by mouth. Additionally, the clinician should take into account the risk of postoperative regurgitation and/or vomiting as side effects of UES myotomy.

Surgical treatment should be considered in patients with severe dysphagia who have not improved after proper rehabilitation treatment.

Appendix

UES Myotomy Combined with Laryngeal Suspension

Physiologically, three main factors are involved in opening the esophageal inlet and allowing a bolus through the UES: relaxation of the UES, pharyngeal peristaltic contraction, and hyolaryngeal elevation. UES myotomy alone is adequate for patients with good pharyngeal contraction. Otherwise, the addition of laryngeal suspension is helpful to compensate for functional swallowing deficiency by achieving the same laryngeal position as occurs during the normal swallowing action.

Indications

1. Failure of a thorough, conservative rehabilitation program, usually lasting >6 months
2. Long-standing history of severe chronic aspiration and recurrent pneumonia (>6 months after onset)
3. Evidence of severe aspiration due to impaired laryngeal elevation, inadequacy of pharyngeal constrictor activity, and/or incoordination and insufficient opening of the esophageal inlet (UES)

Contraindications

1. Overt gastroesophageal regurgitation secondary to a permanently opened esophageal inlet, which eradicates the protective mechanism of the UES against regurgitation and augments the risk of aspiration of gastric contents
2. Cognitive impairment including dementia, mental problems, and inability to follow commands
3. Moderate to severe trunk ataxia
4. Poor general condition

Surgical Procedure

1. UES myotomy
2. Laryngeal suspension surgery. The effect of laryngeal suspension is increased elevation of the larynx. This procedure can be performed using several techniques [15]:
   - *Type 1: Thyrohyoid fixation approach.* This procedure is the simplest technique with which to facilitate upward movement of the larynx by about one vertebral height.
   - *Type 2: Hyoid–mandible fixation approach.* This method is indicated in dysphagic patients with pooling of residue in the vallecula and inadequate epiglottic inversion, which influences laryngeal closure.
   - *Type 3: Thyrohyoid–mandible complex fixation approach.* The thyrohyoid complex is suspended from the mandible, and the infrahyoid muscles are resected. The mandible, hyoid bone, thyroid cartilage, and/or cricoid cartilage are connected by a wire or thread. This procedure is appropriate in patients with UES opening deficits secondary to impaired hyolaryngeal anterior excursion.
   - *Type 4: Thyroid–mandible fixation approach.* This procedure is always performed concurrently with myotomy and is beneficial for patients with severe dysphagia and concurrent suprahyoid muscle weakness. After the operation, the patient must be trained to swallow using a specific swallowing pattern (head extension and neck flexion) to augment the opening of the UES entrance (chin jut) during direct swallowing training (Figs. 8.3 and 8.4).

If oral intake is possible without aspiration by 1–2 months postoperatively, the tracheotomy tube can be removed. Additionally, the functions of mastication and

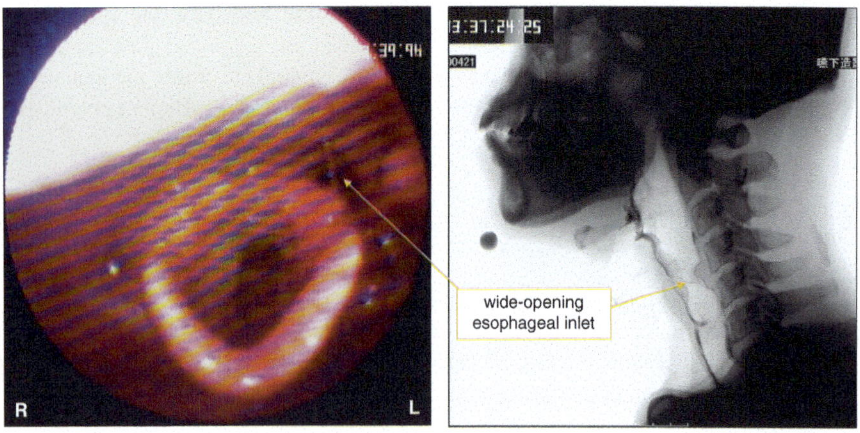

Fig. 8.4 VE and VF images of a widely opening esophageal inlet (UES) following laryngeal suspension and myotomy

tongue movement (which importantly contribute to bolus formation and propulsion) and the presence of pharyngeal residue (which increases the risk of aspiration) should be assessed to determine the patient's eating ability and most appropriate bolus type.

Caution: Respiratory difficulty may occur due to excessive suspension of the laryngeal complex.

References

1. Kisa T, Igo M, Inagawa T, Fukada M, Saito J, Setoyama M. Intermittent oral catheterization (IOC) for dysphagic stroke patients. Jpn J Rehabil Med. 1997;34(2):113–20.
2. Kisa T, Sakai Y, Tadenuma T, Maniwa S. History, application, procedures, and effects of intermittent oral catheterization (IOC). Jpn J Compr Rehabil Sci. 2015;6:91–104.
3. Sugawara H, Ishikawa M, Takayama M, Okamoto T, Sonoda S, Miyai I, et al. Effect of tube feeding method on establishment of oral intake in stroke patients with dysphagia: comparison of intermittent tube feeding and nasogastric tube feeding. Jpn J Compr Rehabil Sci. 2015;6:1–5.
4. Miyazawa Y. Patient Doctors Network: Management of enteral nutrition. 2002. http://www.peg.or.jp/paper/article/nutrition/1-point.html. Accessed 8 October 2016.
5. Davis JW. Prosthodontic management of swallowing disorders. Dysphagia. 1989;3(4):199–205.
6. Gary JJ, Johnson AC, Garner FT. The role of the prosthodontist regarding aspirative dysphagia. J Prosthet Dent. 1992;67(1):101–6.
7. Ohno T, Fujishima I. Palatal and lingual augmentation prosthesis for patients with dysphagia and functional problems: a clinical report. J Prosthet Dent. 2016;117(6):811–3. doi:10.1016/j.prosdent.2016.08.025.
8. Okuno K, Nohara K, Tanaka N, Sasao Y, Sakai T. The efficacy of a lingual augmentation prosthesis for swallowing after a glossectomy: a clinical report. J Prosthet Dent. 2014;111(4):342–5. doi:10.1016/j.prosdent.2013.08.011.
9. Nakayama E, Tohara H, Teramoto K, Nakagawa K, Handa N, Ueda K. A case report of a dysphagia patient treated by palatal augmentation prosthesis. Ronen Shika Igaku. 2009;23(4):404–11. (Japanese)
10. Chieko K. The prosthetic approach for cases with swallowing disorder with dysarthria after brain damage. J Rehabil Sci. 2005;1:91–8. (Japanese)
11. Clinical practice guidelines of PAP for Dysphagia and Dysarthria. Japanese Society of Gerontology and Japan Prosthodontics Society. 2011. (Japanese).
12. Shin T, Tsuda K, Takagi S. Surgical treatment for dysphagia of neuromuscular origin. Folia Phoniatr Logop. 1999;51(4–5):213–9.
13. Fujishima I. Treatment and management for severe dysphagia: medication, rehabilitation and surgery. Rinsho Shinkeigaku. 2011;51(11):1066–8. (Japanese).
14. Mahieu HF, Bree RD, Westerveld GJ, Leemans CR. Laryngeal suspension and upper esophageal sphincter myotomy as a surgical option for treatment of severe aspiration. Oper Tech Otolaryngol. 1999;10(4):305–10.
15. Kos MP, David EF, Aalders IJ, Smit CF, Mahieu HF. Long-term results of laryngeal suspension and upper esophageal sphincter myotomy as treatment for life-threatening aspiration. Ann Otol Rhinol Laryngol. 2008;117(8):574–80.
16. Tomoyuki H. Rehabilitation for dysphagia – think and practice. 2nd ed. Tokyo: Ishiyaku publishers, Inc; 2008. (Japanese)

Part IV
Case Studies

Chapter 9
Case Studies

Yoko Inamoto, Kannit Pongpipatpaiboon, Seiko Shibata, Yoichiro Aoyagai, Hitoshi Kagaya, and Koichiro Matsuo

Abstract This chapter presents three case studies for a more comprehensive understanding of assessment and treatment of dysphagia and discusses common etiologies.

Key learning points in each case study are shown as follows:

Case study 1 and 2

- An appropriate clinical approach in patients with dysphagia is important.
- Physiological abnormalities should be clarified by instrumental evaluation, particularly VF.
- Effective swallowing exercise-based rehabilitation therapies include both element-based exercises and target-oriented exercises.

Case study 3

- The use of various types of instrumental assessments is clinically helpful to obtain more information for kinematic and kinetic analyses. This enhances the understanding of swallowing physiology and helps to establish active therapeutic strategies for the patient.

Y. Inamoto (✉)
Faculty of Rehabilitation, School of Health Sciences, Fujita Health University, Toyoake, Aichi, Japan
e-mail: inamoto@fujita-hu.ac.jp

K. Pongpipatpaiboon • S. Shibata • Y. Aoyagai • H. Kagaya
Department of Rehabilitation Medicine I, School of Medicine, Fujita Health University, Toyoake, Aichi, Japan
e-mail: ning665@gmail.com; sshibata@fujita-hu.ac.jp; yyy@rc5.so-net.ne.jp; hkagaya2@fujita-hu.ac.jp

K. Matsuo
Department of Dentistry, School of Medicine, Fujita Health University, Toyoake, Aichi, Japan
e-mail: kmatsuo@fujita-hu.ac.jp

E. Saitoh et al. (eds.), *Dysphagia Evaluation and Treatment*,
https://doi.org/10.1007/978-981-10-5032-9_9

9.1 Case Study 1

A 59-year-old man had a history of severe right thalamic hemorrhage and respiratory failure 11 months previously. He underwent tracheostomy and did not require a ventilator. He was treated with an antiepileptic drug (sodium valproate, 900 mg/day) continuously after the onset of hemorrhage and respiratory failure, and he had no history of convulsion. He was referred to the Department of Rehabilitation Medicine at Fujita Health University Hospital because of severe dysphagia with multiple recurrent bouts of pneumonia. A nasogastric (NG) tube was placed for nutritional support (Figs. 9.1 and 9.2).

The patient was drowsy and disoriented on admission. Hypersecretion was evident based on the observation of fluid passing through the tracheotomy tube. A weak voluntary cough and drooling were observed. He could tolerate the use of a speech valve for only a short time because of dyspnea. Conjugate eye deviation toward the right side was present. Left hemiplegia and hypoesthesia with loss of proprioception were also observed. Cognitive dysfunction was detected, including left-side neglect, inattention, and memory disturbance. No aphasia or ataxia was noted.

The patient was totally dependent with respect to ADL. His motor Functional Independence Measure (FIM) score, cognitive FIM score, and total FIM score were 16/91, 16/35, and 32/126, respectively.

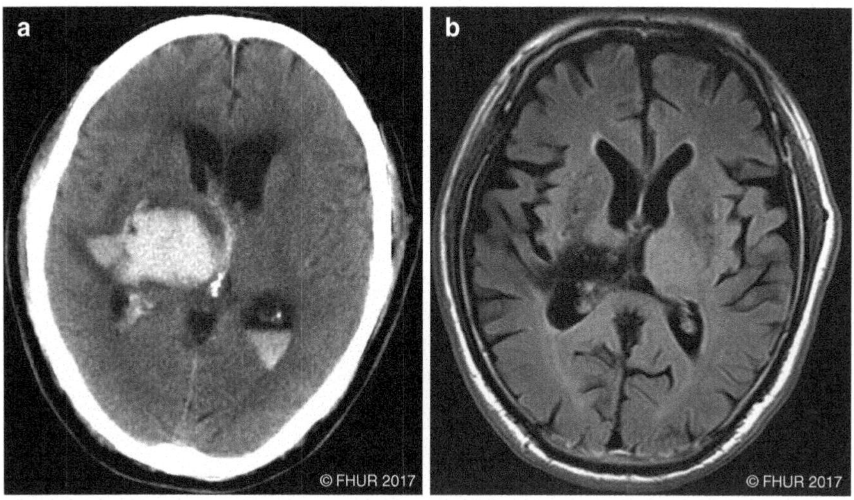

Fig. 9.1 (**a**) Axial CT scan of the brain at the time of hemorrhage onset. The large area of increased density (white) represents acute bleeding in the right thalamic area, and the low density surrounding the blood indicates adjacent cerebral edema. (**b**) Axial fluid-attenuated inversion recovery magnetic resonance image at the time of admission to the rehabilitation ward shows hypointensity involving the right thalamic area

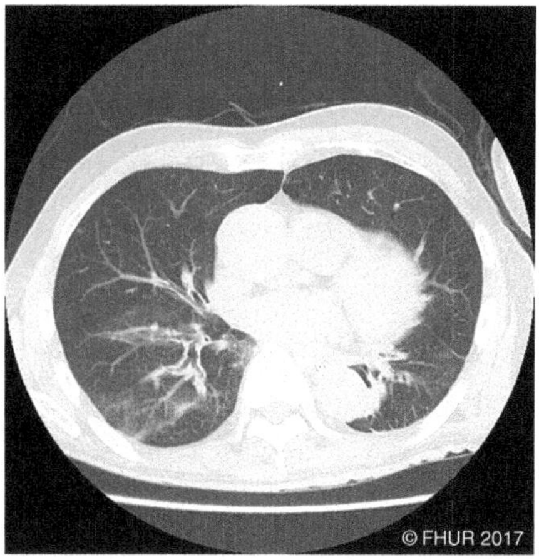

Fig. 9.2 Chest CT at the time of admission to the rehabilitation ward shows bilateral opacities in both lower lungs (more severe on right side), suggesting chronic inflammation secondary to saliva aspiration. The patient had not yet begun oral intake before admission. This sign is crucial to the presence of severe dysphagia

Initial swallowing assessment revealed the following abnormalities associated with the cranial nerves: positive left curtain sign, left tongue deviation, reduced tongue movement in all directions, and weakened oromotor function. Swallowing screening by the repetitive saliva swallowing test (RSST) revealed a score of 2 at admission. Further instrumental examination was recommended to diagnose the dysphagia, clarify the physiological abnormalities, and establish the treatment plan.

9.1.1 Instrumental Swallowing Assessment

VE was performed 1 day after admission. No aspiration occurred during swallowing, and no post-swallow residue using honey-thickened liquid and jelly was observed. However, post-swallow oral residue mixed with saliva was delayed moving downward to the hypopharynx, leading to aspiration. The dysphagia severity scale (DSS) score was 2.

During the next 2 days, the patient was investigated by VF. The VF findings are shown in Table 9.1 and Fig. 9.3).

The first VF study (Table 9.1) showed that the change in the reclining angle had a beneficial effect on bolus control in the oral cavity. The 60° reclining posture contributed to the improvement in oral function by minimizing the duration of bolus manipulation when compared with the 45° reclining posture. All bolus consistencies and textures, including the honey-thickened liquid, nectar-thickened liquid, thin liquid, jelly, and rice porridge, showed the same trend: no penetration, aspiration, or pharyngeal residue in either the pyriform sinus or vallecula. Mild dysfunction of esophageal transition was noted.

The main problems found in the first VF study were the presence of oral residue after swallowing and poor bolus manipulation. Upon returning to the ward, a large

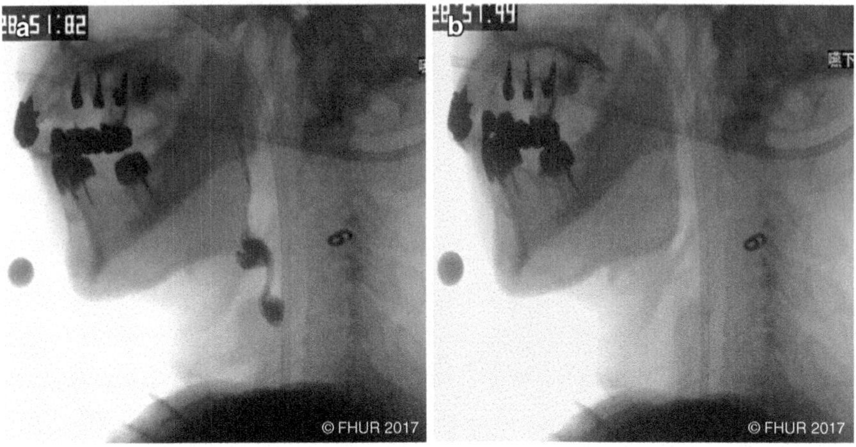

Fig. 9.3 VF using 4 ml of a liquid with honey consistency. (**a**) Impaired bolus formation and inability to propel the bolus from the oral cavity to the pharynx in one swallow. (**b**) Oral barium stasis after swallowing

Table 9.1 VF findings at the initial evaluation

Posture					
View	Degree	Head	Bolus type	Amount of bolus	Findings
Lat	45	N	Honey	4 ml	– Oral residue – Impaired bolus formation and propulsion – No penetration/aspiration – No pharyngeal residue
			Nectar	4 ml	
			Thin LQ	4 ml	
Lat	45	N	Rice porridge	½ spoon	– Oral residue – Prolonged oral stage with slow bolus manipulation and slow mastication – No penetration/aspiration – No pharyngeal residue
During the change of the position to reclining 60°, bolus residue from oral cavity falls late into vallecula and pyriform sinuses before starting the next bolus trial					
Lat	60	N	Honey	4 ml	– Oral residue – Impaired bolus formation and propulsion – No penetration/aspiration – No pharyngeal residue
			Nectar	4 ml	
			Thin LQ	4 ml	
Lat	60	N	Rice porridge	½ spoon	– Oral residue – Shortening the duration of oral stage but still be slow bolus manipulation and slow mastication – No penetration/aspiration – No pharyngeal residue
AP	60	N	Honey	4 ml	– Mild delayed esophageal transition

Degree refers to the angle of the reclining posture

AP anteroposterior, *Lat* lateral, *LQ* liquid, *N* neutral position

Table 9.2 Physiologic abnormalities and other findings at initial evaluation

Stages	Findings	Physiological abnormality
Oral	Oral residue	– Oromotor weakness including tongue and poor coordination
Pharyngeal	– No penetration/aspiration seen during VF test – No pharyngeal residue	– Within normal limit

NOTE: Cognitive dysfunction may affect the results of VF

Table 9.3 Treatments based on initial evaluation

Findings	Physiological abnormality	Functional approach[a]	Postural and diet modification
Oral residue	– Oromotor weakness and poor coordination – Tongue muscle weakness	– Orolingual exercise • Tongue movement exercise • Tongue strengthening exercise • Lip exercise – Chewing exercise	Postural techniques – Reclining 60° Diet modification – Modified food – Thickened liquid

[a]Frequency of rehabilitation: 40 min/time, 1 time/day, 6 times/week

amount of sputum mixed with a barium bolus was suctioned from the tracheostomy tube. This indicated the presence of food aspiration, most likely from oral food stasis after the VF study. Although there was no clear evidence of penetration or aspiration during the VF study, the 10 ml thin liquid, cup drinking, and eating a two-phase food were not tested to ensure safety. Thus, the DSS score was 2 (food aspiration).

Based on the outcomes of VF and VE, the main physical finding was oral residue, and the physiological abnormality was poor bolus control (both bolus formation and propulsion) secondary to orolingual weakness and dysfunction. This resulted in delayed post-swallow aspiration, as mentioned earlier (Table 9.2).

9.1.2 Course of Treatment and Recovery

Initial treatment involved nutritional support, mainly via an NG tube. A SLHT started target-oriented swallowing exercises once a day (lunch time) with nectar-thickened liquid, jelly-type rice porridge, and chopped softened food with thickened liquid at a 60° reclining position. Oromotor exercises including lip exercises, tongue movement exercises (forward-protrusion, left-right side, tongue tip elevation), and tongue strengthening exercises using the Pecopanda tool (JMS, Hiroshima, Japan) were performed as element-based exercises. Additionally, chewing exercises were recommended simultaneously with intensive pulmonary rehabilitation by a physical therapist. Table 9.3 summarizes the treatments performed based on the physiological abnormalities found.

A speech-type valve with a deflated tracheostomy tube cuff was periodically used to control saliva aspiration and perform phonation training. Two days after starting target-oriented training with modified food, the patient developed a low-grade fever without other symptoms, and eating training was temporarily discontinued. Meanwhile, the element-based exercises were continued. The patient's medical condition was generally stable. No increased amount of secretion or leukocytosis was found. The C-reactive protein concentration was slightly rising, however, and a chest radiograph showed mild consolidation in the right lower lobe. The most likely diagnosis was aspiration of saliva, not food. Therefore, the eating training performed by the SLHT was carefully resumed, and the tracheostomy tube cuff was inflated during training. The ward nurse also collaborated with the SLHT to closely observe the patient after meals.

After a 9-day course of swallowing rehabilitation, the antiepileptic drug was stopped; this improved the patient's level of arousal. The patient was able to incrementally increase his cooperate with the swallowing training. His fever gradually resolved along with his improved clinical status, and his blood test results were within normal limits during the following 10 days. In addition, amantadine was started to further promote his swallowing ability (initial dosage, 50 mg/day with a subsequent increase to 100 mg/day in the next week).

The patient's swallowing ability progressively improved, and the NG tube was removed when he was able to ingest three adequately sized meals a day 1 month post-training. Additionally, his secretion status was greatly improved, and the tracheostomy was eventually removed. The RSST score, MWST score, and tongue pressure were 4, 5, and 22.2 ± 2.1 kPa, respectively.

Follow-up VF was performed on day 37 after the first VF study to observe the changes in the patient's abnormal physiology and his response to the rehabilitation treatment (Table 9.4).

Various types of boluses were used during the repeated VF studies to clarify the patient's swallowing ability and clinical improvement. The results showed improvement in his oral function (either bolus formation or propulsion) and decreased oral residue after swallowing. His chewing ability seemed improved compared with the first VF study. However, when chewing food such as corned beef and two-phase food and when drinking a large amount of liquid, orolingual weakness with coordination dysfunction was still observed. Continuation of all exercises was thus recommended with a gradual increase in intensity.

The DSS score was 4 (occasional aspiration). Diet modification was slowly performed in a stepwise manner until ordinary porridge and soft food could be ingested while continuing the nectar-thickened liquid because the risk of thin liquid aspiration still remained. The RSST, MWST, and tongue pressure measurement were repeated, and the results indicated improvements in the swallow ability (4, 5, and 24.8 ± 1.7 kPa, respectively). After 2 months of continuous swallowing training, VF study was repeated.

The results of the third VF study (Table 9.5) demonstrated improved swallowing ability, particularly in bolus manipulation, chewing ability, and orolingual control. The oral residue was still present, although it was decreased. Liquid cup drinking resulted in no deep penetration as detected at the second VF study. The DSS score had changed to 6 (minimum problem).

Table 9.4 Findings of the second VF study (37 days after the first VF study)

Posture					
View	Degree	Head	Bolus type	Amount of bolus	Findings
Lat	90	N	Honey	4 ml	– Reduced oral residue and able to clear by the second swallow – Improved bolus formation and propulsion – No penetration/aspiration – No pharyngeal residue
			Thin LQ	4 ml	
			Thin LQ	10 ml	– Premature spillage – Shallow penetration (PAS 2)
			CB	8 g	– Slightly oral residue – Prolonged mastication, faired bolus formation
			CB + thin LQ	4 g + 3 ml	– Oral residue – Shallow penetration (PAS 2)
			Cup LQ	30 g	– Oral residue – Deep penetration contacting with VFs (PAS 5)
			Straw LQ	30 g	
AP	90	N	Honey	4 ml	– Delayed esophageal transition with slightly esophageal residue

90° refers to the usual sitting-upright position
AP anteroposterior, *CB* corned beef hash, *Lat* lateral, *LQ* liquid, *N* neutral position, *PAS* penetration-aspiration scale *VFs* vocal folds

Table 9.5 Findings of third VF study (59 days after the first VF study)

Posture					
View	Degree	Head	Bolus type	Amount of bolus	Findings
Lat	90	N	Honey	4 ml	– Slightly oral residue – No penetration/aspiration – No pharyngeal residue
			Thin LQ	4 ml	
			Thin LQ	10 ml	– No premature spillage – Slightly oral residue – Shallow penetration (PAS 2)
			CB	8 g	– Shortened the duration of mastication compared with the second VF – Slightly oral residue – Improved bolus formation and propulsion
			CB + thin LQ	4 g + 5 ml	– Oral residue – Shallow penetration (PAS 2)
			Cup LQ	30 g	– Oral residue – Shallow penetration (PAS 3)
AP	90	N	Honey	4 ml	– Delayed esophageal transition with slightly esophageal residue

90° refers to the usual sitting-upright position
CB corned beef hash, *Lat* lateral, *LQ* liquid, *N* neutral position, *PAS* penetration-aspiration scale

The patient's diet was altered in a stepwise manner to soft food, soft rice, and liquid without the use of a thickener. Finally, the patient was able to swallow regular food independently. Therefore, his physiological abnormalities had definitely improved by either spontaneous recovery or the improvement in his consciousness in addition to the effectiveness of swallowing rehabilitation. The progression of the DSS score, eating status scale (ESS) score, and treatment is summarized in Table 9.6.

Eleven months after the onset of hemorrhage, the patient developed recurrent aspiration pneumonia every time he initiated direct exercise; therefore, oral intake

Table 9.6 Progression of treatment and advancements in treatment results

Time[a]	Test	DSS	ESS	Exercises	Recommended diet modification	Recommended posture
Before admission		1	1		No oral feeding	
0	VF	2	2	*Orolingual exercise* – Tongue movement exercise[b] – Tongue strengthening exercise using Pecopanda – Lip exercise *Chewing exercise*	– Paste with small particle – Jelly rice porridge – Nectar-thickened – liquid	Reclining 60°
37	VF	4	5		(Day 37) – Paste with small particle – Rice porridge – Nectar-thickened liquid	Sitting upright
					(Day 44) – Soft food – Rice porridge – Nectar-thickened liquid	
59	VF	6	5		(Day 59) – Soft food – Soft rice – Nectar-thickened liquid	Sitting upright
					(Day 64) – Soft food – Soft rice – Thin liquid	
					(Day 78) – Regular food – Soft rice – Thin liquid	

NOTE: All exercises were gradually increase intensity based on patient condition

[a]Duration (days) after the onset of intensive swallow rehabilitation therapy before admission

[b]Tongue movement exercises consisted of three sets of ten repetitions of each of the following: tongue forward-protrusion-backward, left-right side, and tongue tip exercise

could not be started. However, he achieved the goal of a regular diet 59 days after admission to FHUH. The success of this case illustrates the importance of detailed evaluations of all swallowing components and performance of a systematic intervention. The patient's abnormalities can be summarized as follows:

1. Reduced level of alertness (arousal level), manifesting as low activity due to the use of an anticonvulsant drug
2. Aspiration
   (a) Saliva aspiration due to tracheostomy
   (b) Oromotor dysfunction, especially diminished tongue movement

A transdisciplinary approach is important in swallowing treatment. Symptoms of aspiration pneumonia should be considered as an indication to proceed with treatment. Clinicians must engage in discussions with SLHTs and nurses regarding the patient's symptoms (e.g., fever, amount of expectoration) and whether these are early signs of severe pneumonia or if the patient can continue their exercises, as well as how to adjust the exercise prescription. SLHTs and nurses should regularly evaluate the effects of the swallowing exercises, particularly at the time of step-up. Finally, SLHTs and nurses must always observe the patient for symptoms of aspiration pneumonia and report any remarkable findings to the doctors.

9.2 Case Study 2

A 49-year-old man was diagnosed with acute right lateral medullary infarction at a local hospital and referred to FHUR 1 day later (Fig. 9.4). He complained of swallowing difficulty and the inability to close his right eye. No history of any illness was reported.

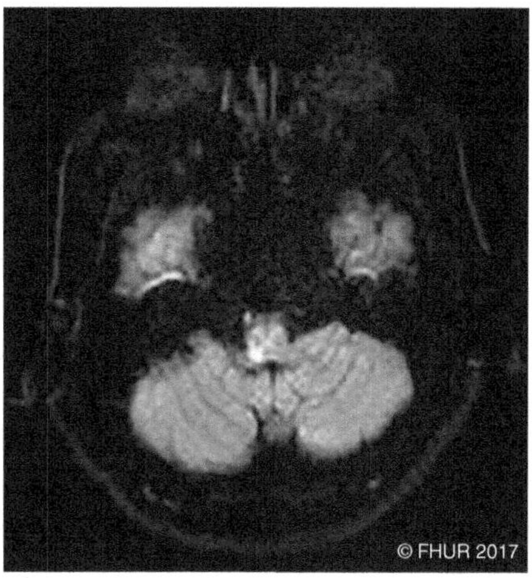

Fig. 9.4 Diffusion-weighted magnetic resonance image showing marked hyperintensity associated with a right-sided dorsolateral medullary infarct

Clinical examination upon admission showed full consciousness with orientation to time, place, and person. Ipsilateral Horner's syndrome and a right curtain sign were observed. Pain and temperature sensations were decreased on the right side of the face and left side of the body. Significant ataxia was present in the right upper extremity, and Romberg's sign was observed. Functional assessment using the FIM showed a motor FIM score of 63/91, cognitive FIM score of 35/35, and total FIM score of 98/126.

Initial swallow assessment revealed that the patient had difficulty swallowing saliva and clearing the throat by expectoration. The tongue range of motion was within normal limits. Swallowing screening revealed an RSST score of 5 and MWST score of 3 (coughing intensely). The patient was maintained at a nothing-per-os status, and a NG tube was inserted for nutritional support.

9.2.1 Instrumental Swallowing Assessment

The initial VE and VF studies were performed 12 days after the onset of symptoms. The VE results showed that a large amount of secretion was present on the pharyngeal wall and in the hypopharynx and could not be cleared by swallowing. No vocal cord paralysis was observed (Fig. 9.5). The DSS and ESS scores were 2 and 1, respectively. Behavioral-based exercises using direct training with special jelly in a safe position (reclining to 60° with right head rotation) was begun thereafter.

The VF study revealed a significant problem in the pharyngeal stage as shown in Table 9.7 and Fig. 9.6.

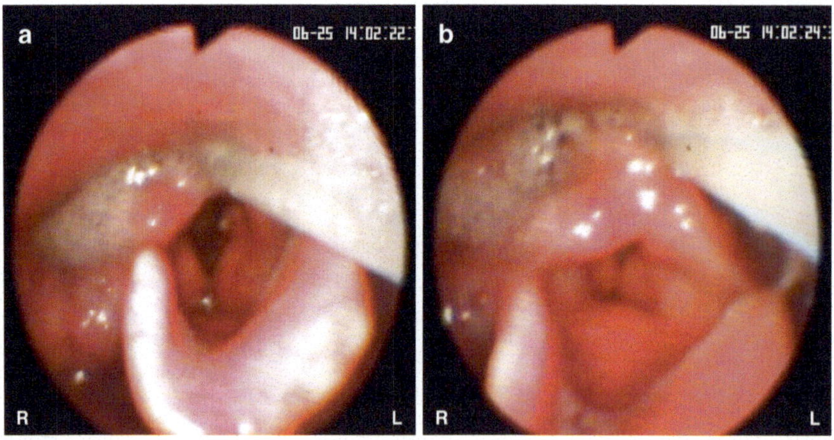

Fig. 9.5 (**a**) A large amount of secretion was present in the hypopharynx and could not be cleared by swallowing. (**b**) Normal apposition of the vocal cords

Table 9.7 Findings of first VF study (12 days after onset of symptoms)

Posture			Bolus type	Amount of bolus	Findings
View	Degree	Head			
Lat	90	N	Honey	4 ml	– Much residue in pyriform sinus – Aspiration after swallowing with spontaneous cough (PAS 7)
Lat	45	N	Honey	4 ml	– No aspiration – Residue in pyriform sinus (able to reduce by repetitive swallows)
AP	45	N	Honey	4 ml	– Bolus passed through Lt UES – Residue in Rt pyriform sinus (able to reduce by repetitive swallows)
AP	45	Rt HR	Honey	4 ml	– Bolus flowed well through Lt UES – No residue
AP	45	Lt HR	Honey	4 ml	– Insufficient bolus flow through Rt UES – Residue in Rt pyriform sinus (unable to enter the esophagus)
Lat	60	Rt HR	Honey	4 ml	– Bolus flowed well through the UES – Decreased residue in pyriform sinus – No aspiration

90° refers to the usual sitting-upright position

AP anteroposterior, *HR* head rotation, *Lat* lateral, *Lt* left, *N* neutral position, *Rt* right, *UES* upper esophageal sphincter

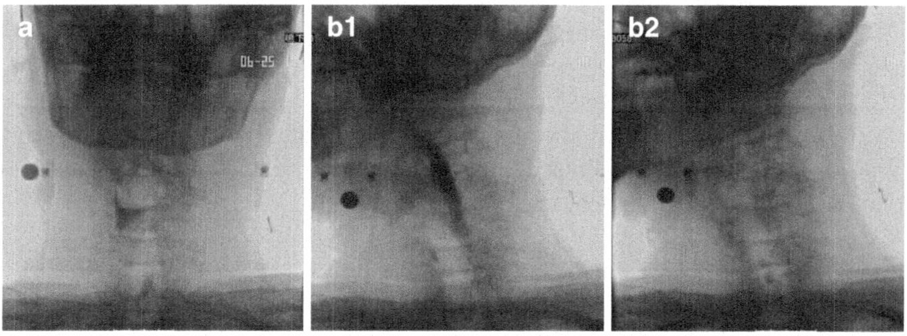

Fig. 9.6 Effect of right head rotation posture during testing with 4 ml of honey liquid. (**a**) Pharyngeal residue is present in the right pyriform sinus after swallowing. (**b**) No residue is present in the pyriform sinus after swallowing when executing the test with right head rotation; b-1 during swallowing, b-2 after swallowing

The VF study was started with the patient sitting upright. Although no aspiration occurred during swallowing, post-swallow aspiration occurred due to a large amount of residue in the pyriform sinus. The examiner changed the reclining angle from 90° to 45° to determine the effect of posture on reducing residue and

Table 9.8 Findings and physiological abnormalities at first evaluation

Stages	Findings	Physiological abnormality
Pharyngeal	– Pyriform sinus residue – Aspiration after the first swallow	– Mild decrease of anterior hyolaryngeal movement – Moderate decrease of pharyngeal constriction – Inadequate UES opening

NOTE: Orolingual function and laryngeal closure were within normal limits

preventing aspiration. The result clearly showed that aspiration was not observed in the 45° reclining posture. Although the residue was decreased by repetitive swallows, it could not be cleared perfectly. Thus, the side on which the residue occurred (laterality) was checked using space manipulation (e.g., head rotation, head/neck flexion) in the anteroposterior view. The results showed that the bolus only passed through the left side of the UES because of paralysis of the right pharyngeal side. Head rotation (space manipulation using the postural technique) was performed to evaluate the applicability, and the residue accumulation was obviously improved more with right than left head rotation. The 60° reclining posture plus right head rotation allowed for safe swallowing without aspiration.

These results indicated that no oral problem was present. The main problem occurred during the pharyngeal stage: a large amount of residue was present, particularly in the right pyriform sinus, causing post-swallow aspiration (penetration-aspiration scale score of 7). The reclining (60°) and right head rotation strategies effectively cleared the residue and eliminated the aspiration. The physiological abnormalities observed from the VF findings are shown in Table 9.8.

Swallow CT was also performed to obtain more details regarding the patient's abnormal pathophysiology, especially pharyngeal constriction and UES opening, which were not easy to evaluate using VF (Fig. 9.7).

The CT outcome, concurrent with the VF outcome, clearly demonstrated that the main physiological abnormalities were pharyngeal constriction weakness, hyolaryngeal excursion, and insufficient UES opening.

9.2.2 Course of Treatment and Recovery

Appropriate treatment was planned based on this understanding of the pathophysiology that was causing the dysphagia (Table 9.9).

As seen in Table 9.7, the posture strategies (reclining posture and right head rotation) and diet modification were effective and could be used to facilitate target-oriented exercises. At the same time, element-based exercises were started, including the Shaker exercise, to improve hyolaryngeal elevation and hence maximize UES opening. The Mendelsohn maneuver was then performed to increase the extension and duration of hyolaryngeal elevation, influencing the augmented UES opening when the patient's condition had improved.

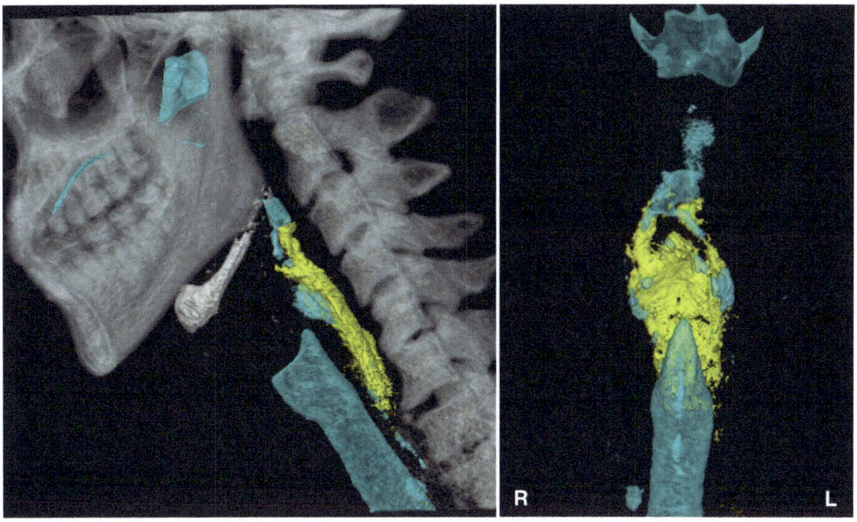

Fig. 9.7 3D-CT images of swallowing 8 ml of nectar-thickened liquid, taken at the time of highest hyoid anterosuperior movement. As the bolus material (*yellow*) passed through the UES inlet during swallowing, air (*blue*) was detected in the pharyngeal space due to pharyngeal contraction weakness

Table 9.9 Summary of treatment based on initial evaluation

Findings	Physiological abnormality	Functional approach	Postural and diet modification
Pyriform sinus residue	– Decreased anterior hyolaryngeal movement – Decreased pharyngeal constriction – Inadequate UES opening	– Shaker exercise – Mendelsohn maneuver – Balloon exercise	*Postural techniques* – Reclining 60° – Rt head rotation *Diet modification* – Modified food – Thickened liquid *Strategies* – 2–3 times of swallow per one bite of food – Clearing throat

Frequency of rehabilitation approach: 40 min/time, 1 time/day, 6 times/week

Because the large amount of pharyngeal residue in the pyriform sinus secondary to UES dysfunction created a high risk of aspiration, balloon dilatation was considered a good treatment option for the patient. The balloon dilatation procedure was thus attempted during the VF study. Although the amount of residue in hypopharynx was reduced, the post-swallow aspiration persisted.

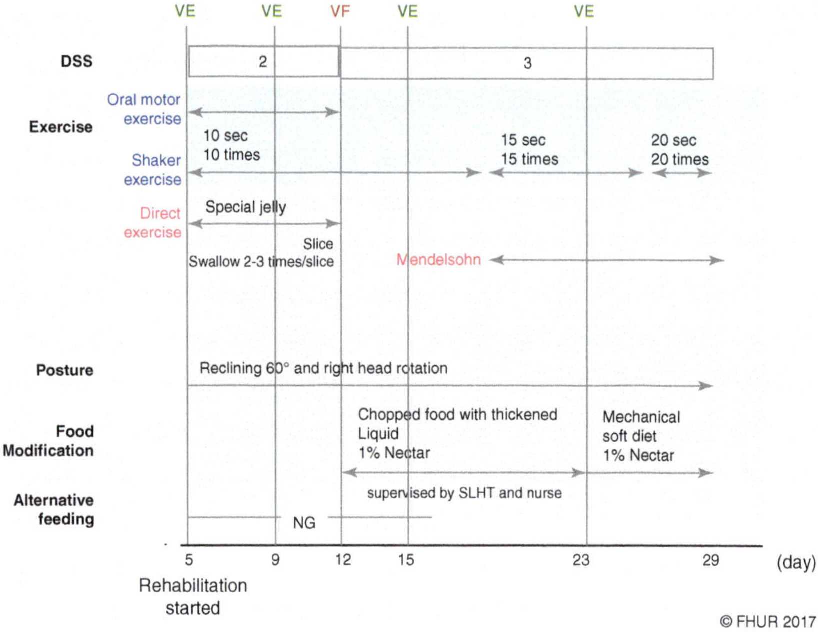

Fig. 9.8 Algorithm of investigation and treatment plan before and after the first VF study with follow-up VE study

This result illustrated the efficacy of the balloon exercise, which was recommended to perform before swallowing exercise to facilitate UES opening during swallow. The patient had no strong gag reflex during insertion of the balloon catheter. Repetitive swallowing and throat clearing were used as strategies during training to reduce the pharyngeal residue.

Chopped softened food with thickened soup, rice gruel, and nectar-thickened liquid were recommended for behavior-based training after VF study. The training was started with one meal a day, and the amount of oral feeding was then slowly increased. VE was repeated to check the patient's clinical improvement, allowing for advancement of the food modification toward mechanical soft food and soft rice. A thickener was still used to prevent aspiration. The NG tube was able to be removed after VE. The DSS score was 3 (water aspiration), indicating no change, but the ESS score had improved from 3 (oral > tube) to 4 (modified oral feeding) (Fig. 9.8).

The VF study was repeated 17 days after the first VF study (29 days after onset of symptoms). After the patient's general condition had improved, the VF study was

Table 9.10 VF findings at the follow-up examination (29 days after onset of symptoms)

Posture				Amount of	
View	Degree	Head	Bolus type	bolus	Findings
Lat	90	N	Honey	4 ml	– No aspiration – Slightly pharyngeal residue (able to clear by repetitive swallows)
Lat	90	N	Thin LQ	4 ml	– No aspiration – No residue
Lat	90	N	Thin LQ	10 ml	– No aspiration – Slightly pharyngeal residue (able to clear by repetitive swallows)
Lat	90	N	Cup LQ	30 g	
Lat	90	N	CB	8 g	
Lat	90	N	CB + thin LQ	4 g + 5 ml	
AP	90	N	Honey	4 ml	– Good bolus flowed through Lt UES

90° refers to the usual sitting-upright position
AP anteroposterior, *CB* corned beef hash, *Lat* lateral, *LQ* liquid, *N* neutral position

performed with the patient sitting upright and with a neutral head position (Table 9.10).

The repeated VF study revealed definitive improvement in swallowing various types of foods and liquids:

1. Decreased residue was present in the pyriform sinus.
2. Aspiration of food of every consistency was eliminated.

Thus, the patient's physiological abnormalities improved, including the anterior hyolaryngeal movement and UES opening.

CT was repeated and revealed increased pharyngeal constriction compared with the previous examination (Fig. 9.9). Additionally, the CT measurement of residue in the pyriform sinus had decreased from 57.5% to 0.6%.

Finally, the DSS and ESS scores at the first and repeated evaluations had increased from 2 (food aspiration) to 4 (occasional aspiration) and from 2 (oral < tube) to 5 (oral feeding), respectively (Table 9.11).

Proper treatment based on all components of a patient's physiological abnormality helps to obtain a positive training outcome. The pathophysiological abnormalities detected by VE and VF must be considered on an individual-patient basis to determine the most appropriate treatment for dysphagia. In the present case, appropriate evaluation, training, postural strategies, and diet modification effectively prevented the development of aspiration pneumonia and improved the patient's eating/swallowing function.

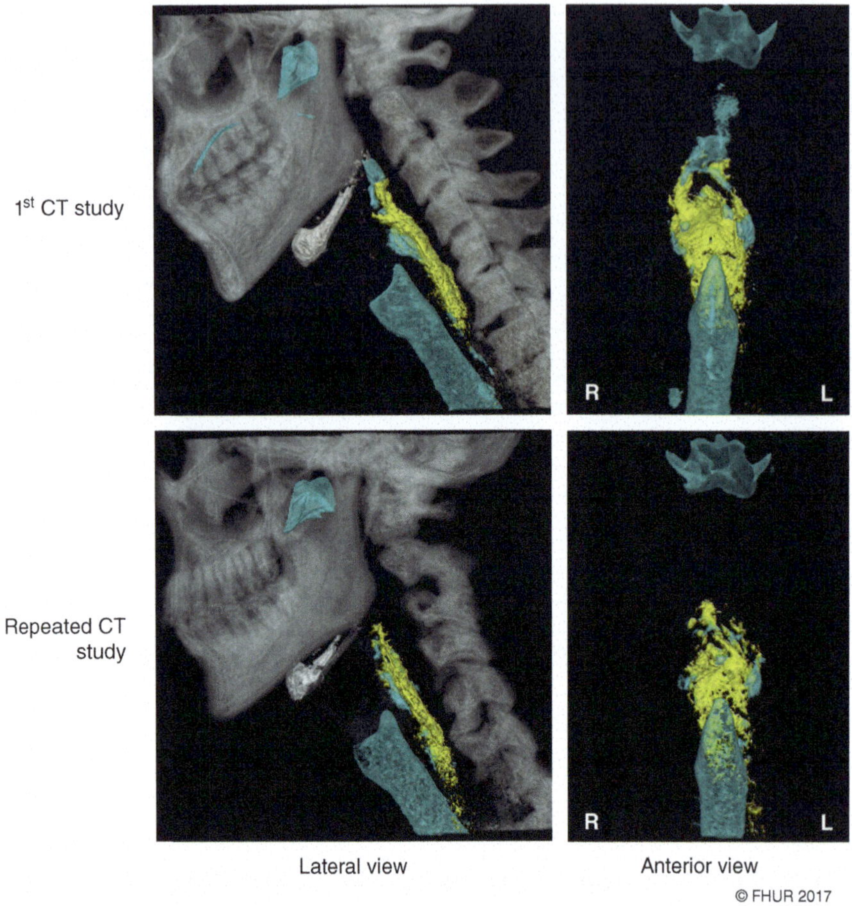

Fig. 9.9 Repeat 3D-CT images of swallowing 8 ml of nectar-thickened liquid, taken at the time of highest hyoid anterosuperior movement. The amount of air (*blue*) in the pharyngeal space while the bolus material (*yellow*) passed through the UES inlet during swallowing was obviously decreased

9.3 Case Study 3

A 75-year-old man presented with left-sided sore throat, neck pain, and a rash of blisters around the left ear and cheek with simultaneous development of acute swallowing difficulty. He was diagnosed with multiple cranial neuropathies caused by varicella-zoster virus infection. VE study revealed multiple white patches on the left side of the soft palate, epiglottis, and arytenoid. The left vocal cord was paralyzed. Although he underwent active treatment after admission, including antiviral and steroid medications, he developed left facial palsy and persistent dysphagia. He

Table 9.11 Summary of treatment progression and advancement of treatment results

Time[a]	Test	DSS	ESS	Exercises and maneuvers	Recommended diet modification	Recommended posture
Before admission		2	1			
5	VE	2	2	– Oromotor exercise – Shaker exercise[a]	Special jelly	Reclining 60° with Rt HR
12	VF	3	3	– Shaker exercise[a] – Balloon exercise	– Chopped food mixed with thickened LQ – Rice porridge – Honey-thickened LQ	Reclining 60° with Rt HR
23	VE	3	4	– Shaker exercise[a] – Mendelsohn – Balloon exercise	– Mechanical soft food (mixed with thickener) – Soft rice – Honey-thickened LQ	Reclining 60° with Rt HR
29	VF	4	5	– Shaker exercise[a] – Mendelsohn	– Regular diet – Soft rice – Thin LQ	Sitting upright (with Rt HR only when having residue feeling)

[a]The intensity of exercise was gradually increased as follows: 10 s of isometric exercise with ten repetitions of isotonic exercise ➔ 15 s/15 times ➔ 20 s/20 times ➔ 30 s/20 times

developed repeated bouts of aspiration pneumonia and underwent percutaneous endoscopic gastrostomy 19 days after the disease onset. He was unable to resume oral intake until referral to the FHUR (135 days after disease onset).

The patient had a history of underlying diabetes mellitus, atherosclerosis obliterans of the lower extremities, atrial fibrillation, and bilateral chronic otitis media. He also had a history of smoking (40 pack-years) and drinking (500 ml of beer every day).

Upon admission, the patient showed a good level of consciousness and no signs of disorientation. There was no acute rash on his face. He had an irregular heartbeat and crackling sound in the left lower lung field. A percutaneous endoscopic gastrostomy tube was placed. The patient also had decreased sensation in the region of the face innervated by the trigeminal nerves (V–III) without any signs of facial palsy or dysarthria. Bilateral hearing impairment was noted.

The patient was partly dependent with respect to ADL. His motor FIM score, cognitive FIM score, and total FIM score were 73/91, 26/35, and 99/126, respectively.

Further investigation by magnetic resonance imaging of the brain showed slight brain atrophy with no remarkable abnormalities.

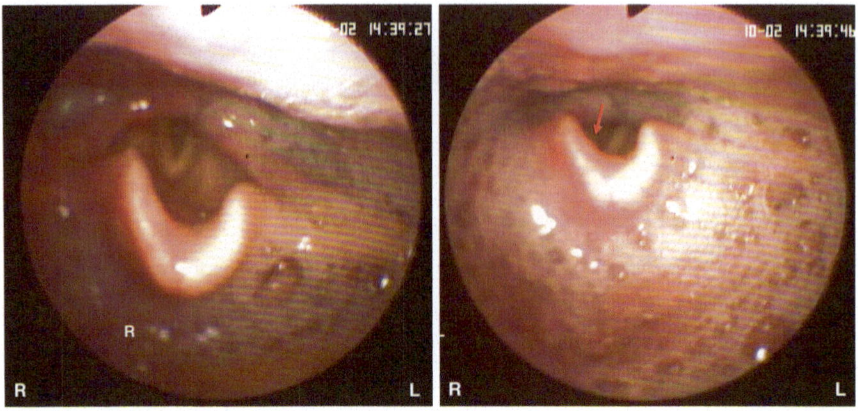

Fig. 9.10 Pooling of saliva in the hypopharynx was unable to be cleared by swallowing, increasing the risk of aspiration into the airway

Initial swallow assessment showed left-sided soft palate paralysis with mild hoarseness. Neither obvious tongue paralysis nor atrophy was observed. Swallowing screening revealed RSST, DSS, and ESS scores of 8 (times in 30 s), 2 (food aspiration), and 1 (tube feeding only), respectively. The tongue pressure at the first measurement was 24.40 ± 2.25 kPa.

9.3.1 *Instrumental Swallowing Assessment*

VE and VF studies were performed after admission (144 days after onset). VE revealed left soft palate paralysis, weakened pharyngeal constriction, and left vocal cord paralysis. Pooling of saliva was present in the pharyngeal recesses and unable to be cleared by swallowing. Saliva aspiration occasionally occurred (Fig. 9.10).

The results of the initial VF study are presented in Table 9.12. The gravity effect was not remarkably different between reclining at 45° and 60°. In contrast to the strategy of space manipulation for the bolus path, right head rotation helped to reduce the amount of residue in the pyriform sinus and reduce the risk of aspiration compared with left head rotation.

However, the residue could not be cleared by only simple postural modification. Many types of boluses were tested at 60° of reclining with right head rotation, indicating that:

- Jelly-type food was helpful to minimize the amount of pharyngeal residue
- Chewed diets (rice porridge and hard jelly) increased the risk of residual aspiration secondary to a low level of swallowing function in the oral and pharyngeal stages

In addition, the modified postural approach, which combines trunk rotation with head rotation, was executed to combine the effects of gravity changes and space manipulation to reduce residue and facilitate safe swallowing. Reclining at 60° combined with left trunk rotation and right head rotation effectively eliminated aspiration and minimized the residue in the pyriform sinus. The DSS score was 3 (water aspiration) (Table 9.12).

Table 9.12 VF findings at the first examination

Posture			Bolus	Amount	
View	Degree	Head	type	of bolus	Findings
Lat	45	N	Honey	2 ml	– Bolus placed in dipper position, need multiple times moving bolus to the dorsum of tongue – Residue in pyriform sinus (able to reduce by repetitive swallows) – No penetration/aspiration
Lat	60	N	Honey	2 ml	– Prolonged oral stage, impaired bolus manipulation with oral residue under tongue – Slight penetration of bolus (PAS 2)
AP	60	N	Honey	2 ml	– Bolus passed bilaterally with much residue in pyriform sinus more on Lt side
		Rt HR	Honey	2 ml	– More residue in pyriform sinus while performing Lt HR with sign of penetration
		Lt HR	Honey	2 ml	
Lat	60	Rt HR	Honey	3 ml	– Oral residue under tongue – Residue in pyriform sinus (able to reduce by repetitive swallows) – No penetration/aspiration
			Soft jelly	Thin slide	– Lessen pharyngeal residue, no penetration/aspiration
			Rice porridge	1/4 spoon	– Slow mastication, impaired bolus manipulation with oral residue – Much residue in pyriform sinus, PAS 2 – Sign of pharyngoesophageal regurgitation
			Hard jelly	Thin slide	– Impaired bolus manipulation, silent aspiration after swallowing from residue in pyriform sinus (PAS 8)
			Nectar	3 ml	– Shallow penetration (PAS 3)
Lat	75	Rt HR	Honey	2 ml	– Aspiration from residue during repetitive swallows (PAS 6)
Lat	60	Rt TR + Lt HR	Honey	2 ml	– Silent aspiration (PAS 8)
		Lt TR + Rt HR	Honey	2 ml	– Easily flow bolus through UES – No aspiration, reduced residue in pyriform sinus

AP anteroposterior, *HR* head rotation, *Lat* lateral, *Lt* left, *N* neutral position, *PAS* penetration-aspiration scale, *Rt* right, *TR* trunk rotation, *UES* upper esophageal sphincter

Table 9.13 Physiological abnormalities and findings of first evaluation

Stages	Findings	Physiological abnormality
Oral	– Oral residue – Impaired bolus holding and manipulation, including bolus formation and propulsion	– Impaired orolingual control: oromotor weakness, including tongue weakness particularly, and poor coordination – Impaired glossopalatal closure
Pharyngeal	– Pyriform sinus residue – Aspiration during swallowing as well as aspiration from bolus residue	– Decrease of anterior hyolaryngeal movement – Impaired laryngeal closure – Decrease of pharyngeal constriction especially on left side – UES dysfunction

The conclusion after the first VF study was that swallowing dysfunction was present in both the oral and pharyngeal stages. Postural adjustment and diet modification effectively prevented aspiration and reduced the pharyngeal residue. The patient's physiological abnormalities based on these findings are shown in Table 9.13.

HRM synchronized with VF was performed for a kinetic evaluation. This examination revealed low bilateral pharyngeal contractile pressure and UES residual pressure, particularly on the left side of the UES (Fig. 9.11).

The HRM results were further supported by electromyography, which revealed patently low muscle electrical activity in the left cricopharyngeal muscle and denervation potential in the left masseter muscle at rest (Fig. 9.12).

Additionally, swallowing CT was performed for quantitative swallowing assessment and showed reduced anterosuperior hyolaryngeal movement (Fig. 9.13).

9.3.2 Course of Treatment and Recovery

A treatment plan was established based on the initial pathophysiological findings.

The main abnormalities in this patient occurred during the oral and pharyngeal stages, as shown in Table 9.14. The patient's impaired orolingual control (including oromotor weakness and incoordination) and glossopalatal closure disorder contributed to the difficulty of bolus holding, formation, and propulsion. Based on the presence of these physiological abnormalities, element-based exercises consisting of oromotor exercises, including tongue exercises as well as target-oriented chewing exercises using Process Lead (Otsuka Pharmaceutical Factory, Inc.), were initiated.

The patient also had multiple pharyngeal dysfunctions resulting in decreases in the anterosuperior hyolaryngeal trajectory and pharyngeal constriction, impaired laryngeal closure, and insufficient UES opening. Based on these results, the patient was prescribed a functional approach involving element-based exercises including the tongue-holding exercise, Shaker exercise, and target-oriented exercises

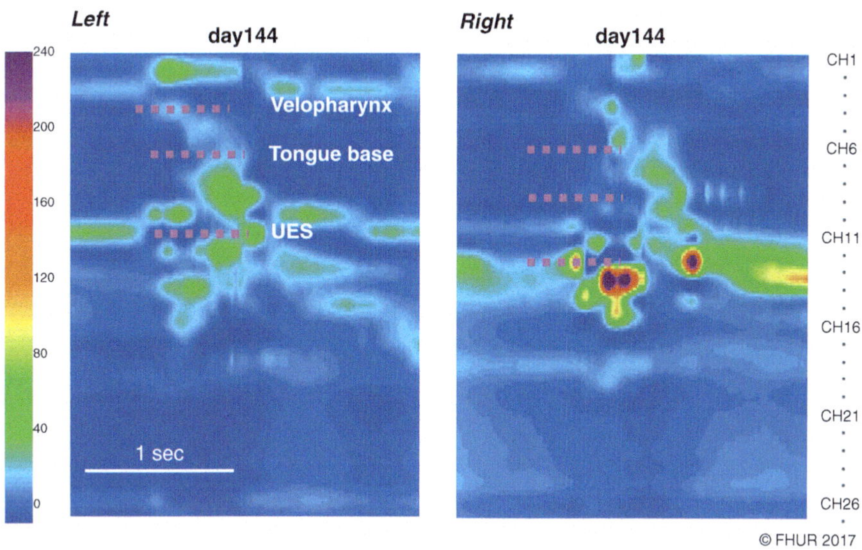

Fig. 9.11 Spatiotemporal pressure tomography plots during saliva swallowing in the neutral head position. Bilaterally generalized low pharyngeal contractile pressure, tongue base pressure, and UES residual pressure, especially on the left side of the sphincter, were present. (*Left*) HRM sensor on the left side. (*Right*) HRM sensor on the right side

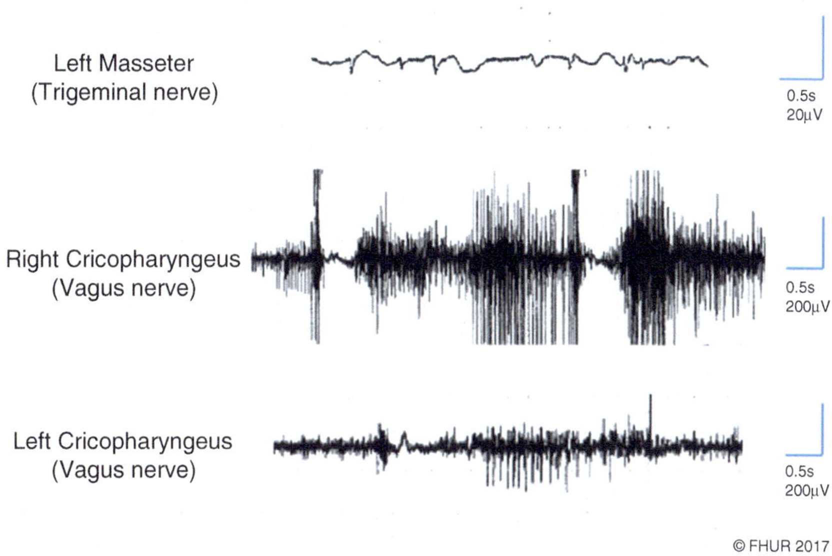

Fig. 9.12 Electromyography signal obtained with a needle electrode from the bilateral cricopharyngeal muscles and left masseter muscle. Left masseter muscle activity was measured at rest. Right and left cricopharyngeal muscle activities were measured separately. Note that the interference pattern and amplitude of the left cricopharyngeal muscle were low

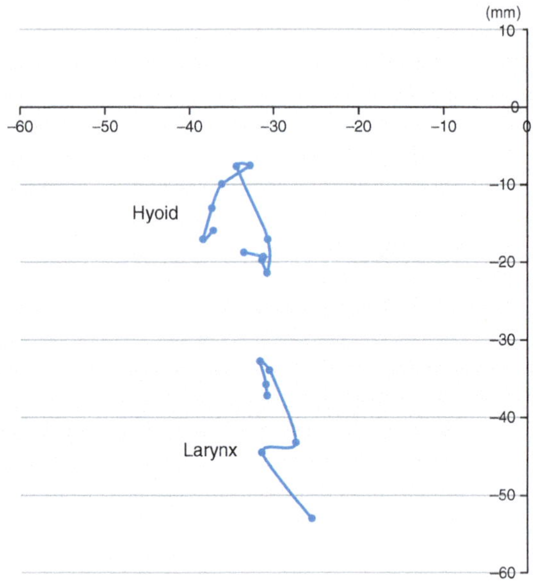

Fig. 9.13 First CT examination (148 days after onset). The graph shows a reduction in the superoanterior hyolaryngeal trajectory (the "0" point is located at the anterosuperior corner of the C4 vertebra)

Table 9.14 Summary of treatment based on the initial evaluation

Findings	Physiological abnormality	Functional approach	Postural and diet modification
– Oral residue – Impaired bolus holding and manipulation	– Impaired orolingual control – Impaired glossopalatal closure – Tongue weakness	– Oromotor exercise – Tongue strengthening and tongue retraction exercise – Chewing exercise	*Postural techniques* – Reclining 60° – Lt trunk rotation and Rt head rotation *Diet modification* – Modified food – Thickened liquid *Strategies* – Repetitive swallows per one bite of food – Clearing throat
Pyriform sinus residue with aspiration	– Decreased anterior hyolaryngeal movement – Decreased pharyngeal constriction – Inadequate UES opening	– Shaker exercise – Tongue-holding exercise – Supraglottic swallow – Mendelsohn maneuver	

Frequency of rehabilitation approach: 60 min/time, 1 time/day, 6 times/week

comprising the supraglottic swallow and Mendelsohn maneuver. The intensity of the exercises was gradually increased, and each type of exercise was started at a different time point based on the patient's condition (Fig. 9.14).

Evaluation of the VF findings allowed for the establishment of a safe functional approach to postural and diet modification. Target-oriented exercise was started once a day at lunchtime by a SLHT using paste food, jelly-type rice porridge, and 2 ml swallows of nectar-thickened liquid. Using the swallowing chair, the patient was placed in the 60° reclining position with left trunk rotation and right head rotation to prevent aspiration and reduce pharyngeal residue. Although the lesion was

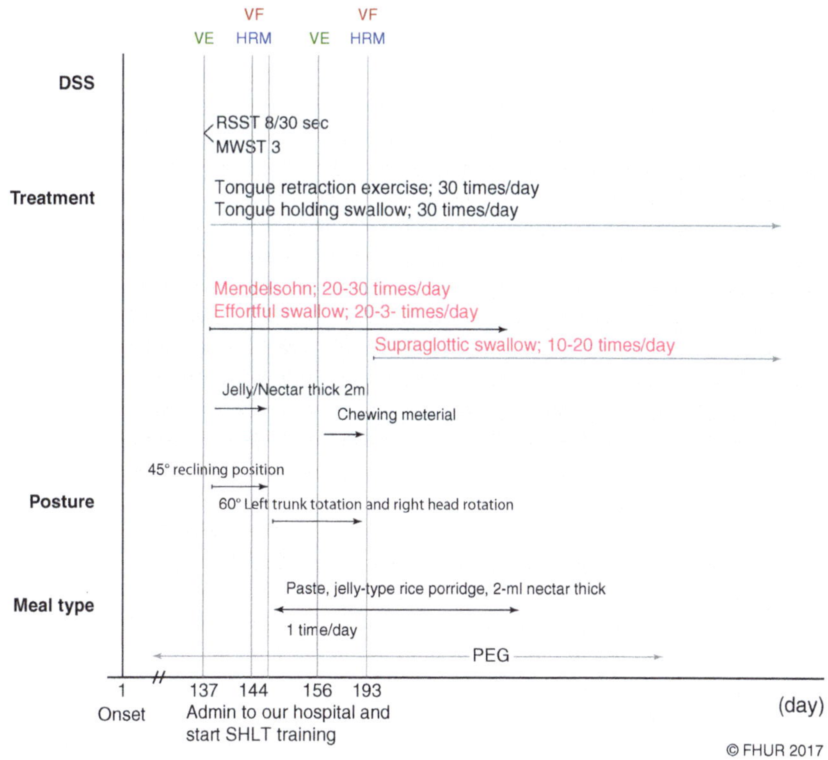

Fig. 9.14 Algorithm of treatment plan, including both element-based exercises and behavioral-based exercises performed concurrently with posture and diet modification, after the initial instrumental evaluations

present on the left side, the risk of aspiration was lower with left trunk rotation and right head rotation, as clearly shown on the VF images. The reason for this might have been the patient's poor laryngeal closure, although his right pharyngeal constriction was functionally satisfactory. In contrast to the more weakened pharyngeal constriction on the left side, the left UES residual pressure was very low due to left vagal nerve palsy, allowing the bolus to easily pass through the UES without aspiration.

The patient's swallowing ability progressively improved. His intake amount was gradually increased during the target-oriented exercises. He showed no signs of aspiration throughout the swallowing rehabilitation period. Follow-up VE, VF, and HRM were executed 193 days after onset to illustrate the improvement in the patient's pathophysiology and reevaluate the treatment plan.

The repeat VE study revealed enhancement of palatal elevation and minimal pooling of saliva in the hypopharynx. The repeat VF study revealed no differences between intake of the honey and nectar boluses or between intake of 3 and 4 ml of nectar. Left head rotation more effectively reduced the pharyngeal residue than did right head rotation when testing with honey in the anteroposterior view; however, no difference was found when testing with rice porridge. A larger bolus volume increased the aspiration risk, particularly with cup drinking and even with the use of the combined postural modification because of the difficulty controlling the posture and volume (Table 9.15).

Table 9.15 Findings of VF at follow-up examination on day 193

Posture				Amount of	
View	Degree	Head	Bolus type	bolus	Findings
Lat	90	N	Honey	3 ml	– Oral residue – Residue in pyriform sinus (able to reduce by repetitive swallows) – Penetration (PAS 3)
		N	Nectar	3 ml	
		N	Nectar	4 ml	
AP	90	N	Honey	3 ml	– Bolus passed both sides, residue in bilateral pyriform sinuses
		Lt HR	Honey	3 ml	– Pharyngeal residue on Lt side
		Rt HR	Honey	3 ml	– More pharyngeal residue in bilateral pyriform sinuses, compared to Lt HR
		Lt HR	Rice porridge	1/3 K-spoon	– Residue in pyriform sinus, mainly on Lt side – Not different between Rt and Lt HR
		Rt HR	Rice porridge	1/3 K-spoon	
Lat	90	Lt HR	Rice porridge	1/3 K-spoon	– Residue in pyriform sinus, PAS 2 – Not different between Rt and Lt HR
		Rt HR	Rice porridge	1/3 K-spoon	
Lat	90	N	Nectar	6 ml	– Oral residue – Silent aspiration (PAS 8); aspiration from residue in pyriform sinus after the first swallow
		Lt HR	Nectar	6 ml	– Deep penetration (PAS 5)
		Lt HR and HF	Cup nectar	30 g	– Oral residue – Silent aspiration (PAS 8), increased residue along pharyngeal wall and in pyriform sinus
		Lt HR	Straw nectar	30 g	– Deep penetration (PAS 5) – Residue in oral cavity and pyriform sinus
		Lt HR	CB	4 g	– Oral residue – Prolonged mastication, impaired bolus formation – Residue in vallecula and pyriform sinus, can't be cleared by repetitive swallows – No penetration/aspiration
			CB + nectar	4 g + 5 ml	– PAS 5

90° refers to the usual sitting-upright position
AP anteroposterior, *CB* corned beef hash, *HF* head flexion, *HR* head rotation, *Lat* lateral, *LQ* liquid, *N* neutral position, *PAS* Penetration-Aspiration Scale

This follow-up VF study demonstrated improved swallowing ability despite the fact that the DSS score (3, water aspiration) had not changed. The patient was able to change his eating posture to the upright position with only left head rotation and neck flexion. The reason for the change from right to left head rotation might have been the strengthening of the right-side (sound-side) structures. Additionally, there was less evidence of penetration and aspiration compared with the prior test, although an increased drinking volume was still associated with a high risk of aspiration. Repeat measurement of the tongue strength revealed an increase from 24.4 kPa to 30.5 kPa.

Follow-up HRM revealed increased tongue base pressure on both sides and increased upper pharyngeal pressure mainly on the left side, as shown in Fig. 9.15.

A follow-up swallow CT study was performed to clarify the improvement in the hyolaryngeal movement (Fig. 9.16).

In addition to the postural change, the patient's diet was altered to rice porridge, chopped softened food with thickened liquid, and continued use of a thickener. The volume was limited to 4 ml for safety. The swallowing exercises were continued.

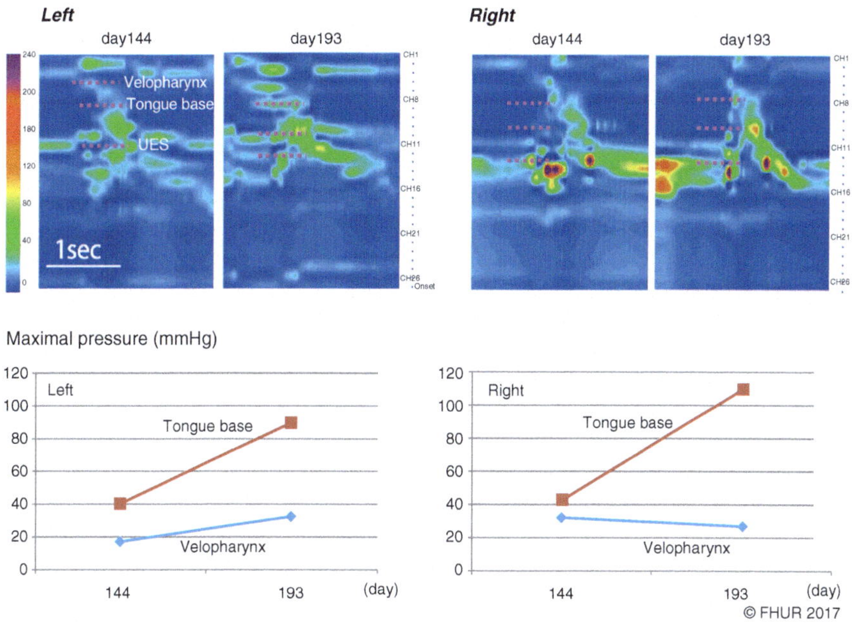

Fig. 9.15 Spatiotemporal pressure tomography plot during saliva swallowing in the neutral head position was repeated after the first evaluation at 7 weeks. The tongue base pressure was improved bilaterally, as was the velopharyngeal pressure (especially on the lesion side). (*Left*) HRM sensor on the left side. (*Right*) HRM sensor on the right side

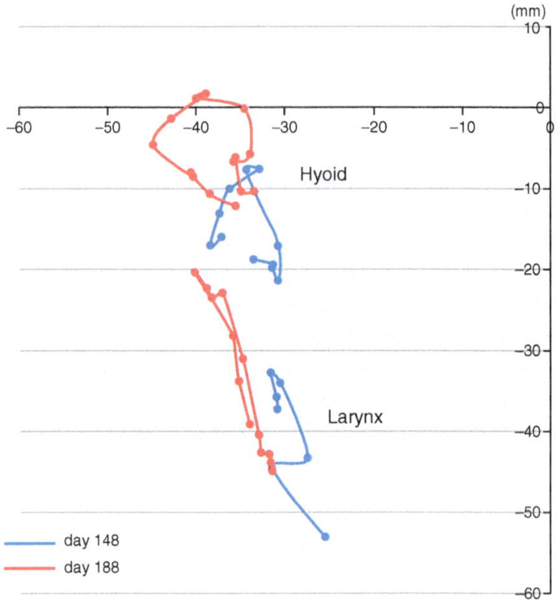

Fig. 9.16 Repeat swallowing CT (183 days after onset) compared with the first computed tomography swallowing CT illustrates improvement in the superoanterior trajectory of the hyoid and larynx (the "0" point is located at the anterosuperior corner of the C4 vertebra)

Table 9.16 Treatment progression and advancement of treatment outcome

Time after onset	Test	DSS	ESS	Exercises and maneuvers	Recommended diet modification	Recommended posture
Before admission		2	1			
144	VF	3	1	– Oromotor exercise – Tongue strengthening and tongue retraction exercise – Chewing exercise – Tongue-holding exercise – Shaker exercise – Supraglottic swallow – Mendelsohn maneuver	– Paste food, jelly-type rice porridge, and honey-thickened liquid	– Reclining 60° – Lt trunk rotation and Rt head rotation
193	VF	3	3		– Rice porridge, paste-type food mixed with small particle, and nectar-thickened liquid	Upright with Lt head rotation

The frequency of meal was increased in a stepwise manner from one to three meals a day under SLHT supervision.

Eventually, the patient's diet was able to be changed to soft rice, soft food with continued use of the thickener, and a limited drinking volume. A summary of the treatment progression and ESS score is shown in Table 9.16.

The percutaneous endoscopic gastrostomy tube was removed before discharge. The patient clearly manifested improvement in his swallowing physiologies secondary to the performance of effective swallowing exercises and spontaneous recovery of the cranial nerves. The target-oriented exercises provided a safe approach, facilitating the improvement in his swallowing physiology.

This patient had a severely complex case of dysphagia that was difficult to treat. In such cases, multiple investigations should be performed for quantitative analysis of both kinematic (e.g., VF, swallow CT) and kinetic (e.g., HRM, electromyography) parameters. An understanding of the pathophysiology of dysphagia based on various types of treatment-oriented evaluations will help clinicians to provide the most appropriate treatment.

Index

E. Saitoh et al. (eds.), *Dysphagia Evaluation and Treatment*,
https://doi.org/10.1007/978-981-10-5032-9

The manufacturer's authorised representative in the EU is Springer Nature Customer Service Centre GmbH, Europaplatz 3, 69115 Heidelberg, Germany. If you have any concerns regarding our products, please contact ProductSafety@springernature.com

Printed and bound by CPI Group (UK) Ltd, Croydon, CR0 4YY
25/09/2026
02222899-0001